Reinventing the Body,

Resurrecting the Soul

On the Shores of Eternity

How to Know God

The Soul in Love

The Chopra Center Herbal Handbook
(with coauthor David Simon)

Grow Younger, Live Longer
(with coauthor David Simon)

The Deeper Wound

The Chopra Center Cookbook
(coauthored by David Simon and Leanne Backer)

The Angel Is Near

The Daughters of Joy

Golf for Enlightenment

Soulmate

The Spontaneous Fulfillment of Desire

Peace Is the Way

The Book of Secrets

Fire in the Heart

The Seven Spiritual Laws of Yoga
(with coauthor David Simon)

Magical Beginnings, Enchanted Lives
(coauthored by David Simon and Vicki Abrams)

Life After Death

Buddha

The Essential How to Know God

The Essential Spontaneous Fulfillment of Desire

The Essential Ageless Body, Timeless Mind

The Third Jesus

Jesus

DEEPAK · CHOPRA

Reinventing the

BODY,

Resurrecting the

SOUL

HOW TO CREATE A NEW YOU

Harmony Books

NEW YORK

All rights reserved.
Published in the United States by Harmony Books, an imprint of the Crown
Publishing Group, a division of Random House, Inc., New York.
www.crownpublishing.com

Harmony Books is a registered trademark and the Harmony Books colophon
is a trademark of Random House, Inc.

Library of Congress Cataloging-in-Publication Data is available upon request

ISBN 978-0-307-45233-7

Printed in the United States of America

Design by Lynne Amft

10 9 8 7 6 5 4 3 2 1

First Edition

To my beloved grandchildren,

Tara, Leela, and Krishan

Contents

Reinventing the Body,

Resurrecting the Soul

INTRODUCTION:
THE FORGOTTEN MIRACLE

In my first semester in medical school, I walked into a stifling dissection room and faced a body lying under a sheet. Pulling back that sheet was shocking—and definitely exciting as well. I took my scalpel and cut a fine line down the skin over the breastbone. The mystery of the human body was about to reveal itself.

At that moment I also stripped the body of its sacred nature. I crossed a line that is nearly impossible to recross ever gain. Thanks to science, a huge amount of factual knowledge has been gained, but at the same time a wealth of spiritual wisdom has been lost.

Why can't we have both?

It would take a leap of creative thinking, a breakthrough. I'm calling this breakthrough the reinvention of the body. You may not realize it, but your body is an invention to begin with. Pick up any medical journal, and you come away with a host of concepts that are purely man-made. One day I sat down and listed the articles of faith I was taught in medical school. It came to a long list of dubious propositions, as follows:

The body is a machine assembled from moving parts, and like all machines it wears out over time.

The body is at constant risk for contamination and disease; a hostile environment teems with invading germs and viruses waiting to overwhelm the body's immune defenses.

Cells and organs are separate from each other and should be studied separately.

Random chemical reactions determine everything that happens in the body.

The brain creates the mind through a storm of electrical impulses combined with biochemical responses that can be manipulated to alter the mind.

Memories are stored in brain cells, even though no one has ever discovered how or where this occurs.

Nothing metaphysical is real; reality comes down to atoms and molecules.

Genes determine our behavior; like microchips, they are programmed to tell the body what to do.

Everything about the body evolved as a matter of survival, the ultimate goal being to find a mate and reproduce.

I used to find this list very convincing. The bodies that I examined and treated in my medical practice conformed to it. Patients came to me with parts that were wearing out. I could pare their symptoms down to treatable problems. I prescribed antibiotics to fend off invading bacteria, and so on. And yet every one of these people lived lives that had nothing to do with machines breaking down and needing repair. These lives were full of meaning and hope, emotions and aspirations, love and suffering. Machines don't lead such lives. Neither do collections of organs. Before long I began to see that the body as seen through the lens of science was inadequate and artificial.

Without a doubt, the body needs reinventing. To have a meaningful life, you have to use your body—you can't experience anything without one—and so your body should be meaningful, too. What would give your body its highest meaning, purpose, intelligence, and creativity? Only the sacred side of our nature. This led me to the phrase "resurrecting the soul." I am hesitant to use religious terms because they are loaded with emotional baggage, but *soul* is unavoidable. Ninety percent of people believe they have a soul, and that it gives their lives ultimate meaning. The soul is divine; it connects us to God. Insofar as life contains love, truth, and beauty, we look to our soul as the source of those qualities; it's no accident that a perfect love is called a soul mate.

There is constant feedback between the soul and the body. We invented the separation between the two, and then came to believe that separation was real.

You may object that you've never felt ecstatic or sensed the presence of God. This simply reflects our narrow conception of the soul, confining it to religion. If you look into the wisdom traditions of every culture, you find that the soul has other meanings. It is the source of life, the spark that animates dead matter. It creates the mind and emotions. In other words, the soul is the very foundation of experience. It serves as the channel for creation as it unfolds in every second. What makes these lofty ideas important is that everything the soul does is translated into a process in the body. You literally cannot have a body without the soul. This is the forgotten miracle. Each of us is a soul made flesh.

I want to prove to you that your body needs reinventing and that you have the power to accomplish that. Every generation has tinkered with the body, strange as that sounds. During the pre-scientific age, the body was deeply distrusted, and it was provided with squalid sanitation, wretched food, and barely enough protection from the elements to survive. Thus it became natural to expect a short, nasty life filled with pain and disease.

So that's exactly what the body produced. People lived thirty years on average, and were scarred for life by childhood illnesses. You and I benefited enormously when this life view became outdated. As we began to expect more from our bodies, we stopped mistreating them. Now your body is ready for the next breakthrough, which will reconnect it with meaning, with the deeper values of the soul. There is no reason to deprive your body of love, beauty, creativity, and inspiration.

You are intended to experience ecstasy just as much as any saint, and when you do, your cells will join in.

Life is meant to be a complete experience. People keep struggling with problems both physical and mental, never suspecting the root cause: that the bond between body and soul has been severed. I wrote this book in the hope of restoring that bond. I'm as eager and optimistic as the first day I used my scalpel to uncover the mysteries waiting under the skin, only now my optimism extends to the spirit as well. The world needs healing. To the extent that you wake up your soul, humankind is waking up the world's soul. It may yet happen that a wave of healing will sweep over us, a small wave at first, but one that could swell beyond all expectations in a single generation.

REINVENTING YOUR BODY

FROM BREAKDOWN TO

BREAKTHROUGH

For you and me, the body poses problems that will only grow worse. As children we loved our bodies and rarely thought about them. As we grew older, though, we soon fell out of love, and with good reason. Billions of dollars are spent to cure the body of its many ills and miseries. Billions more are thrown down the drain for cosmetics, whose purpose is to fool us into thinking we look better than we do. To be blunt, the human body is unsatisfactory and has been for a long time. It can't be trusted, since sickness often strikes without warning. It deteriorates over time and eventually dies. Let's attack this problem seriously. Instead of making do with the physical form you were given at birth, why not look for a breakthrough, a completely new way of approaching the body?

Breakthroughs occur when you start thinking about a problem in a fresh new way. The biggest breakthroughs occur when you start thinking in an unbounded way. Take your eyes away from what you see in the mirror. If you came from Mars and have never seen how the body ages and declines over time, you might believe it would work in just the opposite way. From a biological point of view, there's no reason why the body should be flawed. So start there. Having erased every outworn assumption from your mind, you are now free to entertain some breakthrough ideas that totally change the situation:

Your body is boundless. It is channeling the energy, creativity, and intelligence of the entire universe.

At this moment, the universe is listening through your ears, seeing through your eyes, experiencing through your brain.

Your purpose for being here is to allow the universe to evolve.

None of this is outlandish. The human body is already the universe's most advanced laboratory experiment. You and I are at the cutting edge of life. Our best chance for survival is to embrace that fact. Rapid evolution, faster than that for any other life-form on the planet, gave us our present state of ever-increasing health, longer lifespan, exploding creativity, and a vision of possibilities that science advances faster and faster. Our physical evolution ceased around 200,000 years ago. You don't possess liver, lungs, heart, or kidneys different from those of a cave dweller. Indeed, you share 60 percent of your genes with a banana, 90 percent with a mouse, and more than 99 percent with a chimpanzee. In other words, everything else that makes us human has depended on an evolution that is far more nonphysical than physical. We invented ourselves, and as we did so, we brought our bodies along for the ride.

How you invented yourself

You have been inventing your body from the day you were born, and the reason you don't see it that way is that the process comes so naturally. It's easy to take for granted, and that's the problem. The flaws you see in your body today aren't inherent. They aren't bad news delivered by your genes or mistakes made by Nature. Your choices each played a part in the body you created, either consciously or unconsciously.

Here's a list of physical changes that you have made and continue to make. It's a very basic list, all medically valid, and yet hardly any part of your body is excluded.

Every skill you learn creates a new neural network in your brain.
Every new thought creates a unique pattern of brain activity.

Any change in mood is conveyed via "messenger molecules" to every part of the body, altering the basic chemical activity of each cell.

Every time you exercise, you alter your skeleton and muscles.

Every bite of food you eat alters your daily metabolism, electrolyte balance, and proportion of fat to muscle.

Your sexual activity and the decision to reproduce affects your hormonal balance.

The stress level to which you subject yourself raises and lowers your immune system.

Every hour of total inactivity creates muscle atrophy.

Your genes tune in to your thoughts and emotions, and in mysterious ways they switch on and off according to your desires.

Your immune system gets stronger or weaker in response to being in a loving or unloving relationship.

Crises of grief, loss, and loneliness increase the risk of disease and shortened lifespan.

Using your mind keeps your brain young; not using your brain leads to its decline.

Using these tools, you invented your body and can reinvent it anytime you want. The obvious question is, Why haven't we reinvented our bodies already? Certainly the problems have been staring us in the face long enough. The answer is that solving small pieces of the puzzle has been much easier than seeing the whole. Medicine is practiced in specialties. If you fall in love, an endocrinologist can report on the decline of stress hormones in your endocrine system. A psychiatrist can report on your improved mood, which a neurologist can confirm through a brain scan. A dietician may be worried that you're losing your appetite; on the other hand, what you do eat is digested better. And so it goes. No one can provide you with a complete picture.

To make matters more complex, because the body is so fluid and so superbly multitasking, it's difficult to imagine there's any one step to take that could lead to transformation. Right now you may be in love, pregnant, running down a country lane, eating a new diet, losing sleep or gaining it, doing better at your job or worse. Your body is nothing less than a universe in motion.

Reinventing the body means changing the whole universe.

Trying to tinker with your body misses the forest for the trees. One person fixates on her weight, another trains for a marathon, and yet another is adopting a vegan diet while her friend is dealing with menopause. Thomas Edison didn't tinker with building a better kerosene lamp; he abandoned the use of fire—the only human-generated source of light since prehistoric times—and broke through to a new source. That was a quantum leap in creativity. If you are the creator of your body, what is the quantum leap awaiting you?

Going back to the source

If we use Edison as our model, the last great reinvention of the body followed certain principles:

The body is an object.
It fits together like a complicated machine.
The machine breaks down over time.
The body's machinery is constantly attacked by germs and other microbes, which are also tiny machines on a molecular scale.

But these are all outmoded ideas. If any of these assumptions were true, then the following couldn't happen: a new syndrome recently appeared called *electro-sensitivity*, in which people complain that simply being near electricity causes discomfort and pain. Electro-sensitivity is taken seriously enough that at least one country, Sweden, will pay to have a person's house shielded from the electromagnetic field if they are diagnosed as electro-sensitive.

The widespread fear that cell phones harm the body has reached no definitive conclusion, but it seemed far easier to test whether there is such a thing as electro-sensitivity. In one experiment, subjects were put inside an electromagnetic field (we are surrounded by these every day in the form of microwaves, radio and television signals, cellphone transmissions, and power lines), and as the field was turned on or off, they were asked to say what they felt. It turned out that nobody did better than random. People who described themselves as electrosensitive did no better than anyone else, which means no better than random guessing.

However, this didn't settle the matter. In a follow-up experiment, people were given cell phones and asked if they could feel pain or discomfort when they placed the phones against their heads. The electro-sensitive people described a range of discomfort, including sharp pain and headache, and by looking at their brains with MRIs, it could be seen that they were telling the truth. The pain centers in their brains were activated. The catch is that the cell phones were dummies and were emitting no electrical signals of any kind. Therefore, the mere *expectation* that they would be in pain was enough to create pain in certain people, and the next time they used a real cell phone, they would suffer from the syndrome.

Before you dismiss this as a psychosomatic effect, pause and consider. If someone says he is electro-sensitive, and his brain acts as if he is electro-sensitive, the condition is real—at least for him. Psychosomatic conditions are real for those who experience them. But it's just as true to say that they created the conditions. In fact, there is a much larger phenomenon at work here—the ebb and flow of new diseases that may be new creations. Another example is anorexia and related eating disorders like bulimia. A generation ago, such disorders were rare, and now they appear to be endemic, especially among teenage girls. Premenstrual syndrome, or PMS, had its heyday but now seems to be fading. Cutting, a form of self-mutilation in which the patient, usually a young woman, secretly slices superficial wounds into her skin with a razor or knife, appears to be on the rise after a period of almost total obscurity.

When such new disorders appear, the first reaction is always that the victims created a sickness that is essentially imaginary or psychotic.

Yet when the disorder spreads, and doctors find that patients cannot turn off the switch that turned the illness on, there can be only one conclusion. Self-created symptoms are real.

Machines can't create new disorders. But then the whole machine model was imperfect from the start. If you drive a car long enough, its moving parts are ground down by friction. But if you use a muscle, it gets stronger. Non-use, which helps keeps a machine in pristine condition, leads to atrophy with our bodies. Creaky, arthritic joints seem like a perfect example of moving parts that have worn out, but arthritis is actually caused by a host of complex disorders, not just simple friction.

During your lifetime this outworn model of the body hasn't changed but has only been tinkered with. So what is your body, then, if it's not a machine? Your whole body is a holistic, dynamic process in support of being alive. You are in charge of that process, and yet no one has given you the knowledge of how you should approach your job. Perhaps that is because the enterprise is immense: it covers everything, and it never stops.

The process of life

At this moment your body is a river that never stays the same, a continuous stream merging hundreds of thousands of chemical changes at the cellular level. Those changes aren't random; they constantly serve the purpose of moving life forward and preserving what's best from the past. Your DNA is like an encyclopedia that stores the entire history of evolution. Before you were born, your DNA thumbed through the pages to make sure every piece of knowledge was in place. In the womb, an embryo starts out as a single cell, the simplest form of life. It progresses to a loosely assembled blob of cells. Then, step by step, the embryo goes through the evolutionary stages of fish, amphibian, and lower mammal. Primitive gills appear and then disappear to make way for lungs.

By the time a baby emerges into the world, evolution has overshot the mark. Your brain was too complex as a newborn, with millions of unnecessary neuronal connections built into it, like a telephone system with too many wires. You spent your first few years paring down those millions of surplus connections, discarding the ones you didn't need, keeping those that functioned to make you exactly who you were. But at that point physical evolution reached unknown territory. Choices had to be made that were not automatically built into your genes.

A baby stands at the frontier of the unknown, and its genes have no more old pages left in the encyclopedia. You had to write the next page yourself. As you did so, starting the process of forming a totally unique life, your body kept pace: your genes adapted to how you think, feel, and act. You probably don't know that identical twins, born with exactly the same DNA, look very different genetically when they grow up: certain genes have been switched on, others switched off. By age seventy, images taken of the chromosomes of two twins don't look remotely the same. As life diverges, genes adapt.

Take a simple skill like walking. With each clumsy step, a toddler begins to change its brain. The nerve centers responsible for balance, known as the vestibular system, start to wake up and show activity; this is one area of the brain that can't develop in the uterus. Once a toddler has mastered walking, the vestibular system has completed this phase of its function.

But later, after you grow up, you might want to learn to drive a car, ride a motorcycle, or walk a balance beam. The brain, even though it may be mature, doesn't stop there. Quite the opposite: when you want to learn a new skill, your brain adapts according to your desire. A basic function like balance can be fine-tuned and trained far beyond the base level. This is the miracle of the mind-body connection. You are not hard-wired. Your brain is fluid and flexible, able to create new connections up into very old age. Far from decaying, the brain is an engine of evolution. Where physical evolution appeared to stop, it actually left an open door.

I want to take you through that door, because much more lies beyond it than you ever imagined. You were designed to unlock hidden possibilities that will remain hidden without you. An image comes to mind of probably the greatest feat of balance ever exhibited by a human being. You may have seen photos of it. On August 7, 1974, a French acrobat named Philippe Petit breached security at the World Trade Center. He climbed onto the roof and, with the help of confederates, strung a 450-pound cable between the two towers. Petit balanced himself with a twenty-six-foot pole as he walked out onto the cable, which stretched 140 feet. Both towers were swaying; the wind was high, the drop below his feet was 104 stories, or a quarter of a mile. Petit was a professional high-wire artist (as he called himself), and he had taken a basic ability of the body, balance, to a new stage.

What would terrify a normal person became normal for one person. In essence, Petit was at the cutting edge of evolution. He made eight crossings on the wire, which was only three-quarters of an inch in diameter. At one point Petit sat on the wire and even lay down on it. He realized that this was more than a physical feat. Because of the unwavering concentration that was required, Petit developed a mystical regard for what he was doing. His attention had to focus without allowing fear or distraction to enter for even a second. Normally the brain is totally incapable of such unwavering focus; distractions roam the mind at will; fear automatically responds at the first hint of danger. But one man's clear intention was enough: the brain and body adapted; evolution moved ahead into the unknown.

No more breakdowns, only breakthroughs

You, right this minute, stand at the growing tip of evolution. The next thing you think, the next action you take, will either create a new possibility for you, or it will repeat the past. The areas of possible growth are enormous and yet mostly overlooked. It's worth making a list to see what the territory ahead looks like. I took a piece of paper and wrote down as quickly as possible all the aspects of my life that need growth. I didn't limit myself. Anything I wanted to experience, any obstacle that has been holding me back, any ideal I wanted to live up to went on the list. Here's what I came up with:

Love	Guilt	Eternity
Death	Hope	Timelessness
Transformation	Lack	Action
Afterlife	Faith	Desire
Innocence	Intention	Motivation
Grace	Vision	Karma
Renewal	Selfishness	Choice
Loss	Inspiration	Vulnerability
Insecurity	Power	Illusion
Fear	Control	Freedom
Intuition	Surrender	Presence
Crisis	Forgiveness	Non-attachment
Energy	Rejection	Attention
Trust	Playfulness	Silence
Resistance	Appreciation	Being

If you want to know where the universe wants you to go next, this list offers a lot to choose from. Your soul is funneling energy and intelligence that can be applied in any of these areas. Take love, for example. Today you are either in love, out of love, wondering about love, trying to get more love, spreading your love around, or mourning the loss of love. All of these mental activities, both conscious and unconscious, have consequences for the body. The physiology of a widow grieving for her husband who died of a heart attack is very different from the physiology of a young girl who has just fallen in love. We can measure the differences crudely by drawing a vial of blood and examining hormone levels, immune response, and levels of various messenger molecules that the brain uses to send information to the body. We can get subtler and take an MRI, looking at which areas of the brain light up when a particular emotion is felt. But it's obvious that grief and love are worlds apart, and every cell in your body knows it.

Once you realize how many breakthroughs you'd like to make, the hard part is choosing where to start. Which is why humankind has relied so heavily on great spiritual guides to give us a sense of direction. Imagine that you went to see a new doctor and he turned out to be Jesus or Buddha. If you came in with stomach cramps, Jesus might say, "It's just the flu. The real problem is that you haven't found the Kingdom of God within." After running tests for heart function, Buddha might say, "You have some minor blockage in your coronary artery, but what I really want you to do is get over the illusion of the separate self." In real life nothing close to that happens. Doctors are trained to be technicians. They don't think about your soul, much less work to heal it. A doctor visit is a ritual that's not much different from bringing a car to a mechanic's garage and asking why it doesn't run properly.

Jesus and Buddha didn't leave out any aspect of life. They diagnosed the whole self—physical, mental, emotional, social—with uncanny accuracy. Your soul can take over the function of an ideal physician, because it stands at the junction point between you and the universe. Maybe wherever Jesus and Buddha came from, you can go. The secret is to open yourself up. You never know where the next breakthrough will come. The door opens, and from that moment on, your life is transformed.

Quiz: Are You Ready for Change?

Although we have all lived with outmoded ideas about the body, the momentum of change has been gathering. The old model shows many signs of breaking down. Have you been part of this change? The following quiz examines how receptive you are to personal change. We can all become more open, but it's good to have a starting point before the journey begins.

Answer the following questions:

Yes ___ No __ I believe that the mind influences the body.

Yes ___ No __ I believe that some people have had amazing recoveries from illness their doctors can't explain.

Yes ___ No __ When physical symptoms appear, I seek alternative treatment.

Yes ___ No __ Hands-on healing is a real phenomenon.

Yes ___ No __ People can make themselves sick without a physical cause.

Yes ___ No __ I don't have to see healing to believe it exists.

Yes ___ No __ Traditional medicine knows things that scientific medicine hasn't discovered yet.

Yes ___ No __ I can alter my genes by how I think.

Yes ___ No __ Human lifespan isn't determined by genes.

Yes ___ No __ Scientists will not discover a single gene for aging—the process is far too complex.

Yes ___ No __ Using my brain will keep it from aging.

Yes ___ No __ I have the ability to influence whether I get cancer.

Yes ___ No __ My body responds to my emotions: when they change, so does my body.

Yes ___ No __ Aging contains a major mental component. Your mind can determine whether you age quicker or slower.

Yes ___ No __ I am generally happy with my body.

Yes ___ No __ I don't feel my body is going to betray me.

Yes ___ No __ I pay attention to hygiene, but germs aren't a major issue with me.

Yes ___ No __ I have healed myself at least once.

Yes ___ No __ I've had at least one experience with Eastern medicine (acupuncture, qigong, Ayureveda, Reiki, etc.)

Yes ___ No __ I've used herbal remedies that were effective.

Yes ___ No __ I've used meditation or other stress-reduction techniques.

Yes ___ No __ Prayer has the power to heal.

Yes ___ No __ Miraculous cures are possible and legitimate.

Yes ___ No __ My body has as good a chance of being as healthy ten years from now as it does today.

Yes ___ No __ Even though the average elderly person takes seven prescription drugs, I foresee turning seventy on no drugs at all.

Total Yes _____

Evaluating your score:

0–10 Yes answers. You accept the conventional notion that the body is basically fixed, either by genes or mechanical processes of decay and aging. You expect to wear out over time as you age. Your optimism about alternative medicine is distinctly limited and may be totally overshadowed by skepticism. You would never rely on healers, and look upon so-called miraculous cures as either fraud or self-deception. On the one hand, you trust medical science and expect doctors to take care of you, but on the other, you don't pay much attention to your body and feel fatalistic about things that can go wrong with it.

Given the possibility of a major breakthrough, you feel cautious about making any major changes in your life.

11–20 Yes answers. Your experience has caused you to shift away from conventional wisdom about the body. You are open to change and have broadened your ideas about healing. Either you or your friends have tried some form of alternative treatment with success, and you no longer believe that mainstream medicine is the only answer. Yet the claims of hands-on healing probably make you skeptical. In general, you haven't found a way of understanding the body that's more satisfying than the Western scientific model, yet you are aware that unconventional approaches can be valid.

You are attracted to the possibility of making a major change in your life, although you haven't decided which path is right for you.

21–25 Yes answers. You have made a conscious effort to shift away from the old paradigm. You firmly accept alternative therapies. You seek conventional treatment only after you've tried holistic medicine, and even then you are wary of drugs and surgery. Your view of the body is likely to be tied to a spiritual journey that you take quite seriously. You identify with other seekers of higher consciousness. You believe firmly in hands-on healing. You question whether any form of materialism can really plumb the deeper mysteries of life.

You have embraced personal transformation as a major goal in your life and want to change as rapidly as possible.

Breakthrough #1

Your Physical Body Is a Fiction

Breakthroughs depend on daring ideas, so let's begin with the most daring of all. Your physical body, which you have always assumed to be real, is actually a fiction. If you could see that your physical body is an idea your mind is stubbornly holding on to, an enormous breakthrough would take place. You would no longer be imprisoned in a lump of matter. Best of all, you would be free to adopt a much better idea of your body.

Certainly the five senses seem to confirm our physicality. It might be disturbing to realize that the touch of warm, soft skin is only an idea. But it is. Other cultures have offered very different ideas. To early Christians, the body was spirit made flesh, the fleshly part being an illusion. To touch warm skin was to touch temptation. To the Hopi Indians, the entire universe is a flow of energy and spirit, and therefore the body is a transient event in that flow; to touch warm skin was like touching a puff of wind. Buddhists combine the notions of transience and illusion; to them the body is like a ghostly river, and being attached to it is the source of all suffering. To touch warm skin is to sink deeper into illusion.

Those ideas are just as valid as the idea that you have a physical body—a thing, an object—and they point to a simple fact: there was always something suspicious about human beings fitting so neatly into the material world. Rocks are material, but they don't have emotions. Trees are material, but they have no will. Every cell is composed of matter, but cells don't write music and make art. The universe took human evolution far beyond the physical. Think how strange it would be if you treated a book as merely a physical object. You could burn it for fuel or use it as a doorstop. You could crumple up the pages and play wastepaper-can basketball with them. If the book is big enough, you could hurl it at someone like a weapon. Yet obviously the whole point of a book, its very reason for existing, would be missed. What is a book if not a source of information, inspiration, pleasure, and beauty? It's just as mistaken to approach your body as a physical object, even though it, too, burns fuel, plays games, and turns into a weapon whenever a fistfight or a war breaks out.

Your body already knows that its purpose in life isn't physical. If you look through a microscope and watch a germ being surrounded, engulfed, and destroyed by a white cell known as a *macrophage* (literally, "big eater"), nothing could seem more physical. But your eyes are deceiving you. What you are actually seeing is intelligence at work. A macrophage must first identify the intruder. It must decide if the intruder is friend or foe. Having made this decision, the macrophage must move into close position for attack and then deploy its toxic chemical arsenal for killing the enemy.

Purely physical entities don't make decisions, certainly not such delicate yet potentially fatal ones. If white cells go wrong, a macrophage can start eating the body's own cells, creating an autoimmune disease such as rheumatoid arthritis or lupus, both of which are based on drastically wrong decisions. Yet a white cell's intelligence is so profound that it orchestrates its own death when it is no longer useful. Once it consumes the invading microbe, the macrophage dies, the victim of its own chemical weapons. Its suicide is voluntary and altruistic. A single white cell knows that the good of the many overrides the good of the individual—and so it is that the cell makes the ultimate sacrifice in support of that understanding.

If being physical is an outworn model for the body, moving to a new model is urgent, because how we live is based on our underlying beliefs.

Aiden's story

Some people have already started inventing a new body that isn't based on the old physical model. Aiden is a man now past fifty who is educated enough to have pursued a highly successful career in any field he chose. Instead he went on a spiritual quest that began almost by chance thirty years ago.

"The whole thing started out very normally, with no signs that anything strange was about to happen," Aiden recalls. "I was a typical middle-class kid. I went to college in the aftermath of Vietnam, although I wasn't an idealist or a protester.

"But in my early twenties things began to happen that I had no control over. At night in my sleep I would feel that I was awake. I'd find myself in a kind of bubble that could travel anywhere; when I was in that bubble, it was like leaving my body. I had visions of places I didn't recognize, including fantastic cities and landscapes. I saw people I knew, and felt that I had X-ray vision about their hidden characters. These experiences were incredibly vivid. I couldn't dismiss them purely as dreams, because I sometimes had similar experiences sitting in a chair, only instead of being in a bubble, I'd feel myself rising out of my body. One time I expanded beyond the walls of the room and could see outside my house, watching people and cars go by."

Neurologists would likely label such experiences artifacts of the brain, the kind of sensory distortions created by hallucinogens, epilepsy, and severe mental illness. But whether that's accurate or not, it seems the body's physical limitations can suddenly and unexpectedly disappear. Aiden went on.

"I know now that this kind of experience isn't as freakish as you might think. People have out-of-body episodes all the time. They have visions of angels; they intuit events before they happen. Who hasn't thought of a friend who calls you up on the phone the next minute? But people soon forget these experiences, or dismiss them as tricks of the mind. I went the other way. I took my experiences seriously. I wandered off the map."

We were talking in a meditation center in midtown Manhattan where both of us often saw each other in passing. I knew lots of people with similar stories. Most are fascinated by the prospect of reaching higher states of consciousness. So was he.

"We assume we know what's real and what's not, but the line is much fuzzier than people think," he said. "I saw a news program about a priest in Brooklyn who cures people of chain-smoking. He sits a group of them in his living room and seems to do nothing. But he's going inside and envisions a beam of holy light coming into his body. He asks God to relieve everyone in the room of their smoking habit, and that's it. They walk out and never smoke again. There's a healer in Santa Monica who discovered his calling when a neighbor showed up. She had developed a case of warts that covered her whole body. One night she dreamed that her neighbor could cure her simply by touching her. So she knocked on his door and told him about her dream. He was shocked; he wanted her to go away. But the woman was desperate, and basically to humor her he touched her. Within a day or two every wart had vanished."

Did you see such healing on your own? I asked. Aiden nodded. "Healing exists everywhere, but there's a general level of resistance that keeps people from seeing and accepting it." His conviction was obvious. As for where he is now in his journey, he sees himself as a work in progress.

"I've passed through a lot of phases," he said. "I've chased a lot of ideals and had many disappointments. Did I get close to God? Do I think I'm enlightened? I've stopped worrying about those things."

"What did you learn, then?" I asked him.

"I got put back together. My life isn't confusing anymore. I know that I have a source, and being close to the source is a million times better than wandering around with no clue about who you are."

"So you're the same person who started out on this path?" I said.

Aiden laughed. "I wouldn't even recognize him. Looking back, I can see that I was living in disguise. I took off the mask, and everything changed."

He was talking about self-transformation, a word that has become a cliché, but still has a very real basis. The key to transformation is that you create the change you want to see in yourself (which echoes Gandhi's advice that you must become the change you want to see in the world). In this case, the first changes came in Aiden's body. He wasn't by nature a spiritual seeker. He was probably helped by having no religious or spiritual ideas at all. Having no preconceptions, he was open to change when it came along.

The future of an illusion

Yet change is also a choice. Your body is alive with unknown abilities, but it looks to you for direction. When you introduce a new intention, your body finds a way, on its own, to adapt to anything you want. An example of this has been occurring over the past few years. The younger generation has been developing a brain with new capabilities. Researchers find that children who grow up with video games, iPods, e-mail, texting, and the Internet (so-called "digital natives") generate different brain activity from those who grew up in an earlier generation. Their brains grew sharp in one area—the skills needed to access information quickly and play video games, for example—but dull in other areas that emphasized social bonding and the ability to recognize emotions. If you are the opposite of a digital native (the term for you is "digital naïve"), a week's exposure to playing a video game or using the Internet intensively will stimulate your brain to shape itself to conform to your new digital environment.

Once you change the brain, social norms change along with it. Earlier generations of children learned about the world nested inside a tight-knit family, and so they became social creatures. More recent generations, on the other hand, spend hours a day alone at the computer, and experience a loose-knit family, and often no family at all. They have therefore become clumsy at empathy and social contact. Researchers have known, thanks to a breakthrough now twenty years old, that the brain is "plastic"—adaptable to change, not fixed at birth. Now they face the fact that simple daily activity quickly creates new neural networks. And there seems to be no limit to what the new brain can become.

It can deliver spiritual experiences. In fact, if the brain hadn't created a neural network for tuning in to spirit, there could be no experience of God. It was only in the past few years that medical science caught up with this fact. With the cooperation of His Holiness the Dalai Lama, brain researchers were able to study advanced Buddhist monks who had been meditating between fifteen and forty years. In the laboratory the monks were hooked up to functional MRIs, a type of brain scan that can monitor changes in real time.

The monks were asked to meditate on compassion. In Tibetan Buddhist teaching, compassion is the capacity to help any living creature at any time. As they meditated, the monks began to generate the most intense gamma waves ever seen in a normal brain. Gamma waves are associated with keeping the brain functioning as a whole, and also with higher thinking. The most intense area of activity displayed by the monks was in the left prefrontal cortex, just behind the left side of the forehead. This area is associated with happiness and positive thoughts.

The researchers were elated with their findings, because this was the first time anyone had shown that *mental activity alone can alter the brain.* It was already known that the brain could be trained in its physical performance—athletes, for example, get better the more they practice. We praise them for having talent, will, and courage. All of that may be true. But to a neurologist, the greatest runners, swimmers, and tennis players have highly trained their motor cortex, which is responsible for coordinating the complicated movements needed in any difficult sport. Now it could be shown that the mere wisp of desire—in this case the desire to be compassionate—trains the brain to adapt in the same way.

Mysticism is also at work here. A form of love is holding sway over solid matter. Jesus may have spoken in metaphor when he said that faith no greater than a mustard seed can move mountains, but the force of love can literally move the brain. We were all taught— and have accepted without question—that the brain is a "computer made of meat," to use the brutal phrase from a prominent expert in artificial intelligence at MIT. One piece of hardware, the cortex, is programmed to think, while another, the limbic system, is pro-grammed for emotions. But this hard-and-fast division turns out to be false. If you took a snapshot of the activity in your brain at the very instant you had a great idea, dozens of areas in your brain would be lighting up, and for each new idea, a subtly new pattern would be present. A computer, by contrast, lights up the same circuit boards each time any command is given. The notion of "hard wiring" fits a computer. The brain, which can rewire itself in a split second, is obeying invisible forces totally unrelated to computers.

How, then, can we translate this into everyday life? Experimenters at Harvard have shown the immediate effect of love on the body. Subjects sat in a room to watch a film of Mother Teresa and her work with abandoned children in Calcutta. As the viewers watched the deeply moving images, their breathing rates and blood chemistry changed, revealing greater calm and less stress. These responses are controlled by the brain.

If even a brief exposure to higher love creates a new brain response, what about the effects of love in the long run? Older couples who enjoy a good marriage have been studied, and they report that they love each other more after thirty or forty years than when they first fell in love. But they also report that it's a different kind of love, not the overwhelming infatuation that poets compare to madness, but a steadier, more constant, deeper love. This suggests that like the Tibetan monks, happily married couples are experiencing a change in their brains. There certainly are striking resemblances between the two groups. The monks exposed their minds to a state of calm, openness, peace, and "non-doing," to use a common Buddhist phrase. The brain got used to that unbounded state, and thus it escaped from its own conditioning. Long-standing lovers also experience calm, peace, and openness around each other. Exposure to each other has done the work of meditation.

Subtle action

I've been making an argument that the nonphysical aspect of life is stronger than the physical. Talk of invisible forces may sound overly mystical, but at the personal level we can't disconnect love, a purely invisible force, from the body, and we don't need science to prove that falling in love ignites an intense physical change. Once you stop clinging to the idea that your body is a thing, you realize what should have been obvious: your body is the junction between the visible and invisible worlds. Standing at this junction, you are constantly advancing into new regions of the invisible world. For every new step you take, your body follows.

I call these new steps *subtle actions*, because they involve only the mind, whereas gross actions involve direct contact with the material world. Although subtle action comes naturally to all of us, it can be broken down into steps, as follows:

How Subtle Action Works

1. You go inside and make your intention known.
2. You believe in getting results.
3. You don't resist the process of change.
4. Your body shifts effortlessly at the physical level.
5. You repeat your subtle action until you have mastered the change you desire.

The Tibetan monks accomplished all these steps. They meditated in order to make contact with higher consciousness (Buddhists wouldn't use the word *soul*). They sat quietly, trusting that they would reach their goal. They practiced their discipline diligently, keeping the goal in sight. Through subtle action alone, using no effort or physical struggle, compassion flowed into them. (I am reminded of a famous saying in India that wisdom isn't something you learn, it's something you become.)

If invisible forces really do have power, then a subtle action—one entirely located in the mind—should be able to create even greater change than a gross action. And so it turns out. Subtle action translates into uncanny physical ability. There's another Tibetan meditation called *tumo* that protects the body from the elements. Monks who practice *tumo* can sit in caves overnight at subzero temperatures clad only in a thin silk robe, and at dawn they emerge unaffected. The secret, according to Western medical observers, is that the monks have raised their internal temperature by as much as eight degrees Fahrenheit, a heat that utilizes a specific area of the brain, the hypothalamus. Body temperature is ordinarily an automatic response, yet through subtle action a person can move this response at will.

Biofeedback experiments with ordinary people in the West have followed this example. Subjects are asked to focus on a small patch of skin on the back of their hand and will it to grow hot. Without long practice, many could raise their skin temperature enough, simply through focused attention, so that a red patch appeared on the back of the hand.

Yet Western medicine is baffled by yogic practices in India that go a step further. Yogis have trained themselves in meditation to need only minimal food, barely a hundred calories a day. They have been buried in coffins for days, surviving on tiny amounts of air by lowering their breathing rates and basal metabolism. The most advanced yogis are reputed by Western observers to sit so firmly in *samadhi* (deep awareness) that they cannot be pushed over with physical force.

This doesn't mean that subtle action only works in a biofeedback lab or after years of spiritual discipline. The invisible powers that can be manipulated in such specific ways are everywhere and play a part in every aspect of life. We label them as intelligence and creativity, and see them in action when a white cell devours invading bacteria. Nobel Prizes have been given for figuring out just a fraction of the chemistry involved in immune cells, which turn out to be so complex that now the immune system is known as a "floating brain."

The discovery of intelligent cells did nothing, however, to break down the old model of the physical body. Instead we wound up with a paradox. If a white cell is intelligent, how did it get that way? It's not part of the billions of interacting neurons in the brain. If you are a cell biologist, you must locate a white cell's intelligence in its proteins and enzymes, but those are only simpler molecules linked together, so are simple molecules smart? They are made up of even simpler atoms. Are atoms smart? It would seem quite strange to think that the same carbon we find in a lump of coal is intelligent enough to build a macrophage, along with a handful of other atoms like oxygen and hydrogen.

Should carbon share the Nobel Prize, since it's part of every brilliant brain? Yet you are stuck with this *reductio ad absurdum* unless you want to say that intelligence is an invisible force that white cells happen to express. And that's the very thing a cell biologist—or any physical scientist—cannot conclude, because everything about life, from DNA on up, must have a material basis. How much easier it would be to admit the obvious, that intelligence is an invisible force, one that our bodies use extravagantly. Your body's whole purpose is to join the visible and invisible realms, and intelligence isn't the only force that wants to express itself through you. So do creativity, truth, beauty, and love.

Sometimes it takes a stroke of revelation to bring this home. A man named Damon is returning home to Denver from a routine business trip. Damon steps off the plane expecting to fetch his luggage and take a cab home. Out of the corner of his eye he sees his wife, who has decided to surprise him by meeting him in the reception area.

Damon recalls, "She was just standing there smiling, but in my chest I felt this leap of joy. I don't remember having such a feeling since we first fell in love. It caught me completely off guard, so much so that when my wife walked up, she saw a look on my face. She asked me how I was feeling. I wanted to say 'I love you' more than anything in the world. But I didn't. We had been having problems; she wasn't in the best mood. So I just said I was fine, and we started walking toward baggage claim. But that moment haunts me. I don't know where such intense love came from, but it was so sharp and clear. Sad to say, I never felt comfortable bringing it up again."

Love catches us off guard, because we wander around in a haze of busy activity and predictable events. To have a breakthrough, you must consciously connect with the invisible forces that are everywhere around you, urging you to go beyond your old conditioning. A sudden burst of love must be expressed and acted upon, or else it disappears, and ordinary life takes over once more. Subtle action is urgent and necessary. It invokes these invisible forces and brings them into your body. Once you experience the change that makes, there's no reason to cling to the fiction of being physical any longer.

In Your Life: The Action of Love

Subtle action can make the difference between dreaming of an ideal love and achieving it. In ordinary life, love has become entangled with something else, usually the ego. By nature the ego is selfish, and although love appeals to it, the ego wants to have love on its own terms. These must be sorted out. One person may want to be in control, another to be taken care of. One may feel insecure no matter how much love is directed her way, another may have to dominate his partner in order not to feel vulnerable. But pure love exists, and it can be found. As with everything else, a process is involved. You begin where you are, and you grow through subtle action—that is, you quietly encourage the kind of love you really want.

In your own life, consider the qualities of love at the highest level. The soul's love is

unselfish
giving
blissful
warm and safe
self-sufficient, needing no outside validation
innocent

uncomplicated

kind, compassionate

constant

expanding

comforting

sacred

These are terms you've heard all your life, and you have experienced them either a little bit or a great deal. Sit quietly and summon the memory of one quality, such as kindness, including your memories, visual images, emotions, and people connected with this quality. Stay with your experience for a few minutes. Let it deepen of its own accord. In effect, you are subtly directing your mind to access the quality of kindness, which forms a neural pattern that differs from a mind that doesn't dwell on kindness.

In the same way, you can go within yourself and feel, as completely as possible, what "giving" or "sacred" means to you. Taking one quality at a time, pay attention to it until you have a clear sense of its personal meaning. What moment of love was most unselfish in your past? Can you recapture a sense of innocence, perhaps walking in the woods or gazing at the sea?

Don't try to get through the whole list at one sitting. Return to it every day, and as you do, build up an inner sense of your connection to love. Subtle action works by reaching for a deeper level of awareness. As you become more aware of the love that is inside you, you align with an invisible force. Quietly but steadily, you will find that the higher qualities of love will start to enter your life.

Naturally, you will also be confronted by those times when love has faltered or seemed to leave you out. Face these feelings and memories without avoiding them. This isn't an exercise in happy fantasies. Nor is it necessary to focus on the negative: don't dwell on loneliness, self-pity, anger toward a failed love, or boredom with a current relationship. Many people find it difficult to make this distinction. None of us has been trained in subtle action; therefore we entangle ourselves in all kinds of feelings that we call love, and the result is confusion and needless suffering.

Subtle action sorts out the confusion, gently and effortlessly, by allowing the invisible force of love to make itself known clearly. You stop mistaking other things for it. Here's an example:

Loreen, a young woman from Iowa, moves to a new city to take a job offer. It's a promotion, but Loreen finds herself in a strange setting with none of her old friends. Very quickly she spots a coworker who attracts her interest. Usually she's rather standoffish in relationships, but her initial feelings quickly turn into a deep infatuation. Loreen flirts with this man, who is single and available. He acts friendly, but doesn't ask her out on a date.

She finds that her desire for him is turning into dreams and fantasies. They become more erotic, and she drops stronger hints that she is interested in him romantically. To Loreen's surprise, he says that he knows she's in love with him, but he doesn't feel the same way. He acts sympathetic and understanding, which makes him all the more attractive. Loreen feels torn between her intense desire and the knowledge that he is unavailable. She intensifies her campaign, leaving some suggestive phone messages and lying in wait at work on the off chance that she will "accidentally" run into this man. Things come to a head at the office Christmas party, when she drinks too much and throws herself at him in front of other people. Loreen clutches him so tight that he has to peel her off.

The next day the man leaves a note on her desk advising her to seek help. Loreen feels confused and ashamed. She decides to go to a psychologist. In the first session she describes the situation in tears. "I love him so much, I'm beside myself," she says. The psychologist corrects her. "What you're expressing isn't love." Taken aback, Loreen asks, "If this isn't love, what is it?"

"It's abuse," he says. "You would see that if you didn't feel so desperate. What you're calling love is a mask for deeper feelings you're afraid to face." Loreen is very shaken, but on a deeper level she recognizes the truth in the therapist's words.

People often want to be rescued by love, and thus love gets tied to escapism and fear. Things you are afraid of, such as loneliness, isolation, and not fitting in, must be sorted out and healed on their own, not masked by throwing yourself into a relationship with someone you think will solve your fears for you. People like Loreen usually wind up never facing their neediness. Their brains form a pattern of behavior so familiar that even the most negative feedback doesn't change it. Only subtle action can change the brain by introducing a new intention. (Remember the Tibetan monks and how they became compassionate—a new brain pattern had to be created.) As you learn to heal through subtle action, you won't be forced into situations that promote failure and rejection. Those are reflections of your old inner state, from which you are slowly shifting away.

As negative impressions and memories arise, simply paying attention to them has a healing effect. Subtle action operates by looking, watching, and being aware, but not judging, condemning, or rejecting. The negative imprints of your past are not the real you. They are the scars of experience, whereas the good things from your past are signposts pointing toward an opening. By feeling what love is like inside, you activate dormant impulses of love in the here and now. You signal to the universe that you are open, accepting, and receptive to change.

Then change will appear, first as fresh feelings inside yourself, the fragile sprouting of love in its higher form. Be patient and continue to be aware. More moments will come when you do feel kinder or more unselfish, compassionate, or giving. You will also see reflections of these same qualities outside yourself. You will notice them in other people; they will begin to direct them toward you. Let the process expand. Don't demand kindness or giving of yourself or anyone else. Be like a child again, willing to grow without forcing anything; take a chance, however small, at being vulnerable.

Above all, don't let your self-image stand in the way. Self-image is constructed by the ego. It gives you a façade that you can show the world, but it also turns into a shield behind which you hide. If you let your self-image stand in the way, you can't be open and receptive. Real change requires a relaxed, natural attitude. Sadly, most people expend untold energy in protecting their self-image, defending it from attacks both real and imagined. Instead, take the attitude that there's nothing to protect and nothing to defend. You want to be strong, but true strength comes from love that is certain and self-sufficient. False strength comes from building a wall of self-defensiveness. Keep your focus on feeling what love is like for you, and on gently wanting it to expand.

This is a powerful example of how subtle action can accomplish far more than gross action, because only at the subtle level can you train your brain to be completely new.

Breakthrough #2

Your Real Body Is Energy

It's not enough for a breakthrough to be daring; it must also prove useful. The next breakthrough, which says that your body is pure energy, dramatically passes that test. I can pick up any object—a stick of wood, a match, a tungsten wire—and make it disappear from the physical world. By examining it under an electron microscope, any piece of physical matter turns into a hazy cloud no more solid than fog. It's just another step in magnification for the fog to vanish into pure, invisible vibrations. Releasing the energy in those vibrations is incredibly useful, which is why it changed the world when we humans discovered that wood could be burned, matches could carry fire from one place to another, and tungsten could give off both heat and light when electricity was run through it.

In every case, untapped energy stands at the junction point between the visible and invisible worlds, which is how we've been describing your body. A piece of wood is content to stand at the junction point without doing anything, but your body isn't. Your cells constantly move back and forth across the border, lighting an inner fire. How DNA learned to do this remains a mystery, because it's exactly as if a tungsten wire learned to glow, or a match could strike its own spark, without outside help. But the miracle goes much deeper than that. When wood burns, it crumbles into ashes and is gone. When tungsten incandesces, it is doomed one day to burn out. But DNA grows and multiplies as it releases energy. In fact, the only thing that DNA does is to convert raw energy (heat and electrical impulses) into countless complex processes. And since DNA, like any chemical, is itself made of energy, your body is a cloud of energy keeping itself alive by feeding off more energy.

The closer you look, the more clearly you see that there are mysteries hidden within mysteries here. The India I grew up in was a very

religious country, even more so than today, and it contained a pecu-
liar sort of spiritual groupie, a person who liked to hang around with
saints—*saint* is an honorary term applied to someone in a higher state
of consciousness. Ordinary people hung around them in order to
soak up their energy. As a boy, I had an uncle who was fond of drag-
ging me along on such junkets. At the age of eight or ten I would be
taken to sit cross-legged on the floor, having bowed down and
touched the saint's feet in homage. My uncle would chat with the
yogi or swami, but the real purpose of his visit was to receive *darshan*,
which is the way he soaked up the saint's energy.

As a term, darshan is simple—it basically means "to see" in Sanskrit. But it felt like much more to me: the experience of receiving
someone else's energy was truly wonderful. Certain saints made me
feel buoyant and carefree. Others made my mind go quiet, so that
while I was in the saint's presence, I was at peace. Sometimes the darshan felt unmistakably feminine, as if my mother were smiling at me,
even though the saint was a man (he might have been a devotee of
Devi, the Divine Mother).

I noticed other things from these visits. The effect diminished
with distance. You could be walking toward the saint's hut—these are
generally poor people living in austere seclusion—and step by step,
the closer you got to the door, the more you lost any sense of trouble.
Instead, your mind would become filled with the conviction that God
was in his heaven and all was right with the world. This uplifted state
lasted for a while, but as my uncle drove us back home to Delhi, I felt
less inspired and more my ordinary self, like a battery leaking its electrical charge. After some time, either hours or days, the saint's presence faded into a memory.

People like my uncle weren't just energy junkies. They believed
that exposing themselves to a holy soul (*atman darshan*) raised their
consciousness. For the moment, we don't have to decide if that's valid
or not. But it would be a mistake to call darshan purely mystical.
When you see someone you love, your brain aligns with the love they
have for you, and energy passes between you—that's why the first

flush of love can be so overwhelming. In the New Testament, Jesus not only speaks, but wanders among the people to be seen and touched, and clearly his personal energy has a power all its own.

Think of all the qualities about another person that you intuitively pick up at the energetic level. Besides telling if someone is happy or sad, you can sense whether they feel peaceful or perturbed. Looking into their eyes reveals alertness or dullness, tenderness or indifference. It's hard to think of any human quality that doesn't have a kind of energy "signature." The usefulness of this is that by changing your own signature, you can bring forth any quality you want. Disturbance can be turned into peace, sadness into happiness, dullness into alertness. Your body is an energy converter at a very subtle level, where the most cherished aspects of being alive can be accessed. Saints know full well that they are standing at the junction point between the visible and the invisible, because they feel themselves in the presence of God. The energy they transmit is more subtle than heat or light. It's this same energy that your body is also using in ways that science has yet to fathom.

Energy and health

Consider the most basic function of energy, which is to keep your body alive. Your body is in a healthy state when its energy is in a healthy state. Such a notion goes beyond the worldview of mainstream medicine. A hundred years ago, germs were the stars of medicine. All the excitement centered on discovering new bacteria and viruses, matching them up with the diseases they caused, and then killing the germs before they could hurt the body. Today genes are the stars of the show, and the same pattern is repeating itself. The biggest excitement centers on finding new genes, matching them with specific diseases, then trying to manipulate or splice them before harm is done to the body. Yet the star should have been energy, because germs and genes, like any object, are reducible to energy, and therefore all harm caused to the body is traceable to this fundamental force.

Despite these facts, medicine hangs back from learning more. Energy is too dynamic. It shifts and changes. It leaves few traces behind, and the reason for its myriad changes is poorly understood. By contrast, chemicals are concrete, predictable, and come in small, neat packages. Turned into drugs, they can be handed out to patients in measurable doses. Yet this doesn't get past the underlying truth that drugs, too, are bundles of energy, and the effects they cause in your body (including side effects) are nothing but energy patterns moving one way instead of another. It would be a major breakthrough if we could manipulate the body's energy without resorting to drugs, most of which hit the body too hard and too broadly. If you suffer a bad cut and the doctor injects you with penicillin, the antibiotic goes everywhere in your body. While it's killing germs at the site of your wound, it's also traveling to your intestines and killing the single-celled intestinal flora that enable the digestive process. That's why diarrhea is a common side effect of Penicillin V, the updated form of the original drug produced sixty years ago.

Killing off too many single-celled creatures may seem like a simple action, like too much water overflowing the bathtub, but the chemical effects of penicillin lead to many possible side effects, some on the bizarre side, such as "black, hairy tongue." Others commonly seen include irritation of the mouth or throat, nausea, upset stomach, and vomiting. But you might prove to be hypersensitive to penicillin, and then something alarming can happen, like skin eruptions, fluid in the larynx, and anaphylaxis—this last is a state of sudden shock that can be fatal. The reason for this wide, confusing, unpredictable range of side effects is that energy is complex. Your body is shuffling energy into countless patterns, and when you throw a broadly active drug into the mix, your whole energetic state is affected.

Drugs are powerful and troubling, but everyday actions also alter the body profoundly. When you walk into a room to deliver good or bad news to someone, you may not think that you are manipulating their energy, but you are. Causing someone else to become happy or sad goes deeper than a mood swing: the body is directly influenced, as messenger molecules course through the bloodstream, delivering to trillions of cells the energetic effect of whatever the brain is thinking and feeling. (It's no accident that we say, "The bad news made me sick." Your brain takes in the information, converts it to chemicals, and lets your whole body know if there's trouble in the world. Quite literally, you are metabolizing the news and suffering from the toxins it contains.)

The tiniest change in energy, no more than a few words, can lead to massive physical disruptions. A person may be living happily, only to get the unexpected news that divorce papers have been filed against him, or that his entire bank account has been wiped out. Injecting that information into the body has the same effect as injecting a physical substance: chemical changes occur immediately. Stress, weakness, and decreased functioning will spread from organ to organ. At the very least the person will become depressed, but if the news is devastating enough, normal energy patterns may not return. Grief is a state of distorted energy that can last for years. The loss of a mate can make you more susceptible to disease and shorten your life. (This has been proven statistically among widowers, who are subject to higher heart attack rates and shorter life spans.)

On the surface, heart attacks, early death, depression, and the physical side effects of a drug like penicillin look entirely different from one another. But they have the same root cause: the body's energy patterns are being distorted. It takes only a seed of disruption, such as a single malignant cell, to spread incoherence everywhere; if the seed is allowed to grow, the energy of the whole body will break down. It may sound strange to think of cancer as distorted energy, but that's just what it is. To remove that discomfort, you have to start thinking of the whole body in terms of energy. Dealing with your own energy is the most effortless way to heal yourself, because you are going directly to the source. When a distorted energy pattern returns to normal, the problem disappears. Everyday experience tells us that this is plausible. A small child who thinks that his mother has abandoned him in the grocery store will exhibit multiple signs of physical and mental distress. But when the mother reappears, there is no more cause for anxiety. The normal pattern of feeling loved, wanted, and secure returns. And its return is automatic. The highest healing is equally effortless.

Graham's story

The fact that energy is always creating patterns in, around, and through the body has been incredibly useful to people who can tune in to their own energy.

"At a dinner party several years ago, I saw a guest's hand tremble as he reached for the salt," recalls Graham, a friend of mine in his forties who works as an energy healer. "The man was in his late thirties, and when I asked if something was wrong, he talked freely about having Parkinson's disease. His name was Sam, he owned a small business in town, and he had lived with his diagnosis for seven years. Sam managed his Parkinson's carefully on a minimal dosage of medication, but he knew that was only temporary. Eventually the tremors would worsen, and full-blown Parkinson's would set in."

At the time of this encounter, Graham was just beginning to be interested in energy work. He invited Sam to accompany him to California for a training workshop in an ancient form of Chinese healing called *qigong* (pronounced *chee-GUNG*).

"I was new to any kind of hands-on healing, but I'd always been open to it," Graham said. He had practiced meditation for many years and had read widely in Eastern spirituality. "The notion that the body is composed of subtle energies didn't put me off me the way it does many skeptics.

"My new acquaintance was wary but willing to go with me to the weekend course. When I arrived to drive him to the airport, his tremors were more severe than what I'd seen the first time. We didn't talk about it, though, and the next day we sat in a group of about fifty people who had signed up to learn about qigong."

Qigong, like other traditional Chinese medical treatments, is based on controlling and directing *qi* (or *chi*), the basic life-force that sustains the body. Because some qigong practices are tied to wider spiritual beliefs that are considered non-Communist, qigong in the People's Republic of China has been subject to regulation and sometimes suppression by the government.

"Our teacher, who was from Hong Kong, told us that qi exists at a subtle level of the body. Its natural flow keeps a person healthy, but when these subtle energies get imbalanced, disease results. Generally it takes years of disciplined training to control and change the qi in your body, but our teacher had a new idea, that every thought causes a tiny change in the patterns of qi. He believed that even major illness and trauma could be unraveled, so to speak, by healing tiny mistakes in the qi, one at a time, like tiny links in a chain."

Graham took the training seriously and learned rapidly. Sam was less disciplined; he began with initial excitement, but learned in fits and starts.

"Our teacher brought people up from the audience who had chronic conditions like lower back or neck pain. He made a simple diagnosis, and then he would adjust their qi," said Graham. "The method was simple. In his mind the healer asks if certain aspects of a person are weak or strong. If he gets the feeling that any aspect is weak, he asks for it to go back to being strong, the way it is in a healthy person. These aspects could be anything physical, psychological, or environmental. If you had asthma, for example, our teacher wouldn't ask just about the lungs and respiratory system. He'd ask if the nervous system was weak or strong, he'd look into depression and general fatigue. Any disorder involves hunting for where the chain of energy has broken down, and then repairing it one link at a time. The amazing thing was that the volunteers who came forward with sore backs and necks were healed on the spot."

For many westerners, the story so far contains some unresolved questions. Can the body's energy be detected by someone else? We know what it's like to sense if someone is angry or sad, but we tend to call those emotional states, not energy states. Can we go a step further and call disease an energy state? It's meaningful that cancer is often detected first by the patient, who feels a sudden drop in energy or an unexplained mood shift toward depression or vague uneasiness. Qigong would call this a breakdown in the pattern of qi, while Western medicine waits for more-concrete physical changes before taking action.

Even though we understand in theory that the body's energy patterns are affected at the quantum level, westerners don't recognize that energy can be detected subjectively, either by the sick patient or a healer. The major sticking point in Graham's story, the notion that the qigong healer can change another person's energy through intention, actually fits the field model of physics quite well. In Chinese medicine, qi is a field, just like a magnetic field, and it embraces both patient and healer without any boundaries to separate them. A pocket magnet looks separate and isolated, but it, too, is embraced by the entire magnetic field of the earth.

Graham found that a simple demonstration helped to overcome some initial distrust he had. "In qigong the main pathway of energy is up and down the spine. We got into pairs and did a simple muscle test. While I held my arm straight out, my partner would press down on it. We had no problem resisting the downward pressure on our arms. Then we were asked to envision the energy running down our spines and to follow it in our mind's eye. As soon as I did that, I couldn't resist the pressure on my arm; it became instantly weak.

"Then we reversed the exercise. While my partner kept pushing down on my extended arm, I imagined the energy running *up* my spine. This time it was easy to resist the pressure on my arm; in fact, I felt stronger. At first we used the muscle test with extended arm—a simple form of kinesiology—but after a while the healer could perform the testing in his mind, asking 'weak or strong?' without contacting the patient's body. I know it sounds incredible, but that's the basis of the healing I've been doing for several years now."

And what happened to Sam, the man who suffered from early-onset Parkinson's?

"His tremors decreased dramatically while we were at the course," said Graham. "Sam got very excited and talked about going off his medicine. Driving home from the airport, he seemed like a different person, enthusiastic and totally free of symptoms that I could observe. But I made Sam promise not to go off his medications. We parted, and I don't know what happened after that. I just hope he kept up his qigong practice."

This story isn't just about qigong; it illustrates a larger point: the body is nothing but energy patterns, and whether you are aware of it or not, you are manipulating them. *Energy* is a clumsy word. It doesn't denote how alive the body is, how trillions of cells can cooperate to create a whole, and how, if you increase the positive energy in someone, they become incredibly more alive.

The concept of vital energy hasn't caught on in the West because it leaves no physical traces. Without a map of how this energy flows, comparable to a map of the central nervous system, skeptics can call life energy imaginary. But there are many medical treatments in India and China that rely upon exactly such maps, which were drawn purely by seeing energy channels through intuition. Acupuncture and acupressure are the best known of the Chinese systems.

Here is a story I heard from Henry, a friend who visited a local acupuncturist in Los Angeles. "I had pulled a muscle in my upper arm doing work around the house, and although I thought the pain would go away on its own, it grew worse over the next three weeks. I knew, from doing this sort of thing to myself before, that it was tendinitis. Instead of going to my family doctor, I decided to try an alternative treatment first.

"I was given the name of a good acupuncturist and made an appointment. He said he could help, and as I lay on his table he stuck needles in a few places, not just on my afflicted muscle but also on other places on my neck and shoulder. When the treatment was over and I was about to leave, the acupuncturist surprised me by asking if I was depressed. My mother had died the year before, and I told him that I had been feeling down, even though I didn't think I was still grieving.

"He told me that he had detected weak energy around me. That was how he recognized that I was depressed, and he suggested that I let him do a few things. I didn't want to have more needles in me, but that's not what he did. He pressed a few points along my spine, very gently. He also told me he did a little psychic work at the same time. The whole thing took no more than ten minutes, and he didn't charge me.

"As I was walking back to my car, I couldn't tell if my tendinitis was any better, but my mood had shifted. Suddenly I felt very good. I was buoyant, my footstep was lighter. Only then, when the gray cloud over me had lifted, did I realize that I had been feeling down for quite a while. The next day I was still in a good mood, almost elated. My shoulder improved enough that I didn't go back to the acupuncturist. That visit stands out for receiving a healing I never expected."

The energy to change

The difference between healthy and unhealthy energy can be summarized as follows:

Healthy energy is flowing, flexible, dynamic, balanced, soft, associated with positive feelings.

Unhealthy energy is stuck, frozen, rigid, brittle, hard, out of balance, associated with negative emotions.

You can bring healing to any aspect of your life by shifting an unhealthy energy state into a healthy one. People who can't find a way to change are entangled in one or more of the qualities just listed. The hard, frozen looks of hatred that spouses exchange in a bad marriage express one kind of energy, while the soft, loving looks exchanged in a happy marriage express the other. The distinction between physical and nonphysical is no longer relevant. In your body the soft, flowing blood fats that are healthy can become hard, stuck deposits of plaque in your coronary arteries, which are unhealthy. In society, the soft, flowing exchange between people who are tolerant of each other can turn into hard, stuck feelings of prejudice and animosity.

There are strong indications that energy is more powerful than matter. Studies in longevity, for example, examine why some people live to a healthy old age. Their secret isn't good genes, diet, not smoking, or even exercise, beneficial as all those things may be. The highest correlation for reaching ninety or hundred years of age in good shape is emotional resilience, the ability to bounce back from life's setbacks. That fits neatly with one of the qualities of healthy energy: flexibility.

Starting in the late 1940s, Harvard Medical School undertook a study of young males to see why some developed premature heart attacks in middle age. The leading correlation wasn't high cholesterol, bad diet, smoking, or a sedentary lifestyle. The men who escaped premature heart attacks were likely to be those who faced their psychological problems during their twenties, as opposed to men who ignored them. Psychological problems are marked by stuck, rigid attitudes and distorted emotions, pointing us once again to the importance of energy.

I know a woman with a hair-trigger temper who recently received a joke video that was going around, the kind that inserts your name into a generic scenario. It was voting season, and the video was titled "The one person who caused the election to be lost." It showed a mock newscast about how the presidency had been lost because a single voter had stayed home on election day. Her name was inserted into it. Most people would see this as a harmless reminder to vote, but this woman became incensed. She wrote angry e-mails to the organization that was circulating the videos, condemning them for invading her privacy. It was hours before she stopped fuming, and for most of the day her family knew to stay out of her way.

Here we see every sign of unhealthy energy in action. She was already stuck in a pattern of getting angry. Her outrage was rigid and unyielding. It took a long time to subside, and it was associated with negative emotions (not just anger but resentment, victimization, and self-pity). Once she had erupted, it would do little good to treat the outward manifestations. Assuring her that the video was just a joke, imploring her to be reasonable, placating her with distractions or cheering up would all have missed the underlying cause, which was energy-based.

Mainstream medicine vaguely understands how negative emotions can bleed into physical symptoms. But two problems have blocked this from being a fruitful road to treatment. First, distorted energy is too general and widespread. It isn't possible to define a "cancer personality," for example, because disease-prone people are open to all kinds of disorders; there's no one-to-one match between anxiety, for example, and cancer. Finding a simple correlation between negative thinking and a single disorder hasn't worked out, either; nor can being generally positive in your thinking safeguard you from a particular disorder. Your risk factors will improve overall by a certain percentage (usually small) compared with negative people, but beyond that, statistics don't give us any answers.

Second, having detected unhealthy energy patterns, conventional medicine isn't equipped to offer a cure. Psychiatry comes the closest, but it is slow and unpredictable—traditional talk or "couch" therapy can last for years. Taking a shortcut by giving a drug, typically for anxiety and depression, alleviates the symptom but doesn't cure the underlying disorder. The effectiveness of a pill ends the day you stop taking it. Still, psychiatry does direct us to the region of energy where words and thoughts are powerful enough to move molecules. To give just one instance, Prozac, the antidepressant that launched the era of billion-dollar drugs, had an unexpected side effect: it proved effective in treating obsessive-compulsive disorder (OCD).

Patients suffering from OCD look like perfect examples of people whose lives are run by their brains. They cannot stop repeating the same behavior (hand-washing, cleaning the house, adding up the numbers on license plates), and their minds are filled with obsessive thoughts that return no matter how hard the person tries to evict them. Using a brain scan, neurologists can spot an abnormality in such patients—specifically, low blood flow to the orbitofrontal cortex. This region is associated with being able to make decisions and behave flexibly, the very thing OCD sufferers can't do well.

Prozac restores normal activity in the brains of OCD patients, and with that finding, neurology moved a little closer to seeing the brain as an all-purpose chemical factory that determines behavior. But then a new discovery threw that view into question. When OCD patients seek so-called couch therapy, it turns out that talking through their problems can also relieve their symptoms, and brain scans reveal that normal activity has been restored to their brains, only without a drug. This makes logical sense as well. If you are depressed about losing your money in the stock market, taking an antidepressant may relieve your symptoms, but having the market shoot back up will do the same thing, and far more effectively, because now you may have a reason to be euphoric.

Our ingrained habit in this society is to grab the Prozac and bypass the psychiatrist, which once again comes down to trusting the physical over the nonphysical. We must overcome this bias, but how? Does this mean we should all immediately seek psychotherapy?

Most studies indicate that we are becoming by the decade a more anxious and depressed society, more hooked on antidepressants and tranquilizers. Stress levels keep increasing, whether from loud noise, long work hours without rest, interrupted sleep patterns, or pressure at work. Anyone suffering from such stressors will tend to show a marked imbalance in the body, such as elevated blood pressure, increased stress hormones like cortisol, or irregular heart rhythms. Psychiatry can't address such a wide swath of problems. Trying to create a patch of coherence in someone's life does small good when their whole system is in chaos.

What's really needed is a broad-spectrum cure. If all the qualities of unhealthy energy, from blockages and rigidity to negative emotions, could be healed at once, your body could quickly rebound to its natural state of health; it already knows how to thrive in the flow of healthy energy. It takes one more breakthrough to find such a cure, which we will come to next.

In Your Life: How Efficient Is Your Energy?

Every life-form uses energy with great efficiency. A wolf, leopard, or field mouse instinctively knows what food to eat, where to find it, how to survive hardship, and how to obey the rhythms of nature. Animals use life energy in the optimal way for their species.

Unlike creatures in the wild, you and I can manage our supply of energy any way we choose. How you employ your energy makes all the difference between a life well lived and one that is squandered. You and I parse our energy according to the way we express emotions, intelligence, awareness, action, and creativity, since all of these aspects require subtle energy. Much more than burning calories is at stake. Energy must be considered holistically, because when body and soul are aligned, every aspect of life is affected.

To get a better idea of what energy efficiency means, take the following profile quiz. For each item, rate yourself from 1 to 3 according to how well it describes you.

3 - This is how I am ***almost all*** the time.
2 - This is how I am ***some*** of the time.
1 - This is how I am *a **little*** of the time.

___ I leave work on time every day. I don't stay late more than one day a week.

___ I get up and go to sleep at the same time every day.

___ My desk at work is organized. There's not a big backlog.

___ I don't procrastinate. I believe that the best way to handle unpleasant tasks is to face them right away.

___ I don't harbor negativity for a long time. Keeping score and waiting for payback isn't my style.

___ My closet is organized. I can get at anything I want easily.

__ My refrigerator isn't full of leftovers. I'm not surprised by old fruits and vegetables I forgot I had.

__ I know where I stand emotionally with the people in my life. We are open and clear with one another.

__ I know my weaknesses and have a plan for overcoming them. I will be stronger tomorrow than I was yesterday.

__ I use money well. I don't hoard and I don't spend recklessly. I am not worried about my credit card balances.

__ My salary fits my needs for now and the future. I am a good financial planner.

__ My yard is maintained in all seasons. (If you don't have a yard, substitute patio, balcony, house plants, or personal environment.)

__ I keep up with my housekeeping. I'm not faced with accumulated dust and dirt that's piled up for weeks.

__ When I go shopping, I come back with what I need. I rarely have to run back because I forgot something.

__ I keep up with how everyone in my family is doing. I have a good idea of what's going on in their lives.

__ I don't have to rush at the last minute to get things done. I am good at scheduling and balancing my time.

__ I feel that there's a good balance between work and play in my life. I'm having fun and getting things done.

_____ *Total Score*

Looking at your score:

43–51 points. You are leading an efficient life and have a good chance of feeling comfortable, contented, and in control. There are no drastic imbalances in how you use your time and energy. Each aspect of your existence is given a good amount of attention.

36–42 points. Your life is mostly under control and runs along well

enough. You have minor areas of neglect, however, and there are times
when you feel a little overwhelmed by all the things left undone. If you
look closely, there are aspects of your life where you know you could be
more efficient, using your time and energy better. Attending to those
aspects now will increase your sense of comfort and contentment.

26–35 points. Your life is inefficient. You have a sense that you
are treading water rather than getting ahead. Too much is out of your
control, and your ability to cope with everyday challenges is only ade-
quate. To begin to feel more comfortable, you will have to discipline
yourself and change your habits. Look realistically at your inefficient
ways, because sloppiness or disorganization, procrastination or denial,
impulsiveness or neglect drain our energy.

17–25 points. Your life is barely your own because so much is out
of your control. Daily life is a struggle just to keep things together,
and most days you feel that you are losing that fight. On the periph-
ery something very wrong is probably happening. You are being held
back either psychologically or by bad circumstances. To get back on
track, outside professional help will be needed.

As you can see, energy gets diverted into dozens of areas in your life.
When people find themselves struggling, they are squandering their
energies. Two solutions are available: you can increase the flow of subtle
energy into your life, or you can use what you have more efficiently. The
best way to increase your supply of subtle energy is to stop blocking it.
The best way to use the energy you have more efficiently is to expand
your awareness. The great secret of awareness, as we saw, is that it can
accomplish anything while doing almost nothing. The model for the
body is always the soul, and the soul uses no energy at all. We'll go
deeper into this by seeing how subtle energy gets blocked and distorted.
At this point just be aware that you can receive more of the boundless
energy your soul has to offer, and put it to good use in your life.

Breakthrough #3

Awareness Has Magic

We need a breakthrough to manage the body's energy. If distorted energy is the root of all problems, how can it be brought back to its normal, healthy state? No one has taught us how to move energy. We are left to operate on the physical plane, which is not only too crude but very often beside the point. One reads medical articles, for example, that reduce love to a chemical reaction in the brain. The neural activity of someone in love certainly looks different on an MRI from that of someone who isn't in love—specific areas light up, and there are changes in the levels of key chemicals like serotonin and dopamine, which are linked to feelings of happiness and well-being.

Yet it's totally false to say that the brain creates love. Imagine yourself sitting in a car late at night. Beside you is someone you have secretly loved, but you've masked your feelings, unable to express what's in your heart. She (or he) leans over and whispers something in your ear. Whether the words are "I love you" or "I don't love you" will make all the difference. An MRI machine, if it happened to come along on our date, would detect a completely altered state of your brain depending on whether the words make you feel elated or dejected. Yet it's obvious that the brain didn't create these states on its own. The words did. How? They made you aware of something you desperately wanted to know.

In other words, you became aware of whether or not you are loved. Words, when spoken into someone's ear, vibrate air molecules that in turn vibrate the tympanum, sending a signal to the inner ear and on to the auditory region of the cortex. That chain of events would happen even if the words were in a foreign language, yet unless you understand the language, your awareness won't change. Awareness is where meaning happens. If you want to change your body, a change in awareness must come first.

Awareness acts like an invisible force, the most powerful one in your body. It moves energy while seeming to do nothing. Here we have the breakthrough we needed, because awareness can turn unhealthy energy into healthy energy entirely on its own. That is its unique magic.

David's story

There are many mysteries to how awareness works. Let me begin with one that affects everyone's life, the mystery of seeing. When you see something, you become aware of it, and that alone can be enough to move the body in a completely new direction.

David, who is now in his thirties, was born a twin, but he had a tiny genetic heart defect that his twin lacked. "I was lucky, and my heart was repaired soon after I was born," he relates. "There was no reason for me to be treated any differently from my brother. But I remember from early on my mother's anxious looks whenever I tried to do anything she thought was risky. My brother didn't get those looks, and by the time we were four or five, he was considered the strong one while I was the sensitive one. My family members, on the male side at least, are all outdoor types. If you hunted and fished, you got approving looks. If you stayed indoors and read books, you got indifferent or worried looks.

"There's a lot more to raising kids than looking at them, of course. My parents did their best to provide equally for us and to love us the same way. I accepted that I was the fragile twin, and as we grew up, it amazed me how wrong my parents had been. My brother didn't turn out to be a great success. He holds a low-level company job, and since his real passion is hunting and fishing, that's what he concentrates on. I, who always expected to be on the sidelines, grew up to get scholarships, a much better education, and a teaching job at a good university.

"It took me years to realize that we were both shaped to become what we are. If my mother had accidentally switched us in our cribs one day, I would have been the hunter and fisherman, my brother would have become the scholar. It gives me real pause. What went on during those first three years before I have any memory? My parents looked at me in a certain light, and as a result the raw material of an infant got molded one way instead of another."

This is one example of seeing, but many others come to mind. We look at those we love entirely differently from people we don't love. If someone close to us does something wrong, our gaze usually contains sympathy, tolerance, and forgiveness that isn't directed to someone we don't love—they may receive accusation, judgment, and hostility instead. Your gaze doesn't fall passively. It conveys meaning; it makes another person aware of something. In other words, your awareness speaks to theirs, and that is enough to create changes in the brain, leading to changes elsewhere in the body.

There's no limit to the result. Violence can break out on the streets when one male eyes a female the wrong way—according to the male who thinks she's his. (In the Southern United States, there was a long period when an innocent glance by a black male could lead to a lynching.) The secret is to create positive effects instead of negative ones. It's a mistake to believe that you are some kind of radio telescope passively receiving signals from the universe. Seeing is active. You send out energy, and take in energy from others. You can decide to see with love and understanding, acceptance and tolerance. When you do, these qualities exert a force on your surroundings that benefits everything and everyone.

Body awareness

Awareness would have no power if the body didn't respond to it. But think of how massive those responses actually are. If you feel a suspicious lump under the skin, a visit to the doctor will tell you that you are either all right or in danger. If you are in danger, the threat could be mild or severe. Each is a state of awareness ("I'm okay, there's nothing to worry about," "I'm in trouble," "I'm not safe," "I may not make it"), and each brings a sharply different reaction. Even if we say that the reaction is psychological, such as depression in the face of bad news, there has to be a physical response: altered brain chemistry supports what's happening in the psyche. In fact, your body is aware of everything. Every cell knows what your brain is thinking, how your moods change, where your deepest beliefs lie. As your awareness changes, your energy changes, and then your body changes. The chain of events moves from the invisible realm to the visible on this path:

$$\text{AWARENESS} \longrightarrow \text{ENERGY} \longrightarrow \text{BODY}$$

Simple as this diagram looks, it maps a profound breakthrough, because it explains medical findings that are otherwise mysterious. For example, nobody understands a result from the Helsinki Study, one of the most famous research projects in preventing heart attacks. Middle-aged Finnish men at high risk for heart disease were divided into two groups. One, the casual group, visited their doctors a few times a year and were given general advice about losing weight, exercising, improving their diet, and not smoking (advice they were unlikely to follow, given that they hadn't in the past). The other group was followed intensively and put on a specialized program to reduce specific heart-attack risks such as high blood pressure and elevated cholesterol.

At the end of the study, the researchers were stunned to see that the casually followed group had not only fewer deaths overall, but fewer deaths from heart attacks. How could that be? A commentator on the study remarked that it might be a health risk to constantly worry about your heart and see that worry reflected by a doctor you visit too often. From the level of awareness, this explanation makes sense. It also makes sense of many diverse findings along the same lines. The fact is that men who confront their psychological problems in their twenties are doing more to prevent early heart attacks than if they reduced their cholesterol. Elderly people who are emotionally resilient have a better chance of living a long, healthy life than do elderly patients who are less resilient but take vitamins and get regular checkups. Such findings are only a mystery if you ignore awareness and energy, the two foundations of the body.

Millions of people don't make this connection, and they are doomed to fight against their bodies. Think of the whole area of addictions and cravings. To someone who can't stop gaining weight, it seems that a physical craving is forcing them to overeat. Instead of normal hunger, they feel an urge to eat that goes beyond. But in fact the physical impulse masks what's actually going on. The body has gotten stuck in a distorted pattern of behavior that began in awareness.

What happens when you feel a craving? You are torn in two directions: the impulse to resist fights the urge to give in. Let's say you get up at midnight and pad downstairs to the refrigerator because you crave ice cream. At that moment, as you waver over eating a carton of double chocolate chip royale, you may resist the urge, but you won't change your habit. Your awareness is warring against itself. Engaging in this conflict, which happens over and over for people who overeat, gives a bad habit its power, because all your energy goes into fighting against yourself with very little going toward a solution. If the solution existed at the level of struggle, one side or the other would prevail. Either the craving would conquer your resistance, or your resistance would conquer the craving, but the result is a seesaw instead.

It's hard to look past your physical craving, because bad habits always create a groove that the body follows over and over. The craving doesn't have to be for material things like the sweet taste of ice cream or the energy jolt of cigarettes. You may be in the habit of flying off the handle or fretting over every little thing. Anger and worry feel just as physical as hunger. People who crave power or money describe it as being almost sexual. People who crave winning describe it as a burst of adrenaline-fueled elation. Your body mirrors your desires so skillfully, completely, and silently that tracing the chain of events back to awareness isn't easy. But we have to do it if we don't want to be prisoners of our cravings.

We all possess a level of awareness that doesn't crave anything at all. It stands apart from the struggle over "Do I eat this whole carton of ice cream or don't I?" When you find yourself at this level of awareness, the energy to eat isn't activated, and when there's no energy, the body doesn't act. Everyday experience validates this—when someone is grieving, for example, the appetite for food vanishes. The same is true in cases of depression or deep worry, or when we're falling in love. "I can't think about food at a time like this" is frequently heard at such times, and it's accurate: your awareness can't focus on eating, therefore there's no energy behind it, and your body stops feeling hungry. The problem is that just as energy can get stuck in unhealthy patterns, so can awareness, which is why so-called "emotional eaters" have been conditioned to respond in exactly the opposite of the normal response: they overeat in times of grief, depression, and worry.

Your body needs you to master how awareness works. Your state of mind sets the physical agenda in trillions of cells, and they have no power to overturn the agenda on their own. Here's what mastery of awareness looks like.

When You Are Fully Aware

You can center yourself at will.

You are familiar with a place of peace and silence inside.

You aren't divided against yourself by inner conflicts.

You can transcend local disturbances and remain unaffected by them.

You see the world from an expanded perspective.

Your inner world is organized.

This is what it means to rise above cravings. As you start to dip your spoon into the carton of double chocolate chip royale, your body doesn't instantly find the same old groove and your mind doesn't start struggling between "Do I, or don't I?" Instead, other ideas are free to come to mind. "Am I doing this because I'm upset?" "Is this how I really want to handle my situation?" "What has ice cream got to do with getting the stress out of my life?" These are the kinds of ideas that liberate you from any craving. You see what you're doing, and that gives you space to back away. Seeing is never far away when somebody is truly aware; blindness is never very far away when someone isn't.

Once a craving has dug a deep enough groove, it's much more difficult to change your habitual response. (We all know what it's like to take the first bite of a tempting food and blank out until the last bite is gone—the body has taken over completely.) A psychologist would use the word *conditioning* to describe such a well-worn groove. Old conditioning keeps us from being free, because time and again we fall into patterns that run too deep, while our new behavior, the one we wish we could have, has no groove to follow at all. This state of being trapped in old conditioning creates its own kind of awareness.

When Your Awareness Is Conditioned

You can't find your center, so impulses pull you this way and that.

You aren't familiar with a place of peace and silence, so there's constant restlessness.

Conflicting impulses fight against each other.

Local disturbances disturb and distract you.

You see the world from a contracted perspective.

Your inner world is totally disorganized.

We all know at some level that being conditioned limits our lives and stands between us and fulfillment. Consider how the term "unconditional love" came to be so popular. When people seek unconditional love, they want to transcend love as it usually exists, which is highly conditioned: it's restless, unreliable, easily distracted and disturbed; at any moment this love can fall prey to jealousy, anger, boredom, betrayal, or simply a whim if a more attractive love object comes along. Yet we have an intuitive sense that love without conditions must exist—traditionally God's love fulfilled this wish, but now the search is more profane. We want to love a real person unconditionally, and be loved unconditionally in return.

This desire isn't realistic if you look at human nature under ordinary circumstances. It becomes realistic if awareness can shift out of its old conditioning, however. If you can reach a state of unconditional love for yourself, you will be in a completely new energy state, and you find yourself free to love anew. Awareness has the power to deliver unconditional love, and it does so through the same means as putting an end to a craving for ice cream: you see how to transcend your old, unhealthy conditioning.

Three ways to end conditioning

Once you understand how conditioned you actually are, the desire arises to regain control of your life, because every conditioned habit is like an automatic switch that sets a fixed behavior. What sets these switches in place? Time and repetition. Your body adapts to things you do over and over again. It's much easier to set an energy pattern than a physical one, and once set, it's much harder to change.

For instance, if you take up running on a regular basis, you can train an out-of-shape body to run a twenty-six-mile marathon in three to five months. With time and repetition, meaning regular runs of two to ten miles, your body adapts to the agenda you've set for it. You've deliberately conditioned it. On the day after the marathon, if you stop running, your body will be out of shape within a year, usually within half that time. (One research study found something even more drastic: if college athletes in the peak of fitness are put flat on their backs in a hospital bed and not allowed to get up, within two weeks their muscles lose ten years of training.)

Compare those factors with mental conditioning. A single traumatic event (a severe auto accident, being the victim of a crime, living through a terrorist attack) alters your awareness immediately, much faster than physical conditioning. Once imprinted, the mental trauma keeps repeating itself obsessively—images, thoughts, and feelings roam through your mind involuntarily—and those patterns become difficult to change. The most dramatic example is drug addiction, because the mental component that drives someone to use drugs remains in place even when the body has been cleared of toxic substances.

There are three ways to break down old conditioning: reflection, contemplation, and meditation. Their power increases in that order. We all tend to use those words interchangeably, but they have separate implications.

Reflection—taking a second look at old habits, beliefs, and assumptions.

Contemplation—focusing on a thought or image until it expands as far as it can.

Meditation—finding the level of the mind that isn't conditioned.

We aren't interested—not for the moment, at least—in the spiritual significance of these practices. Our primary concern is whether they are effective in moving stuck energy and changing old conditioning. It turns out that their efficacy is very different, and contrary to what you might expect, the more focused you are about attacking a specific energy pattern, the *less* likely you are to succeed in getting rid of it.

Reflection involves standing back and taking a look at yourself, as if in a mirror. It's the same as having second thoughts or reconsidering a past moment in a more settled state. Let's say you have a sudden impulse (to tell off your boss, walk out on your spouse, ask a beautiful woman for a date), but then reflect on whether it's really a good idea or not. Reflection calls upon experience; it lends caution to snap judgments. As a way of breaking down old conditioning, reflection works if you can see something in a new light.

Carla, a woman in her early forties, recounted such an experience. "I grew up in the rural South, and although my family were all
nice people, they had a set of fixed beliefs that everyone seemed to
absorb from the air or the drinking water. My parents didn't consider
themselves prejudiced, yet they had only white friends. They didn't
strike up chats with a waiter or store clerk except white ones. The
small talk I grew up around was knee-jerk conservative, and from an
early age I chafed at hearing it.

"By the time I went to college I was the outsider. I worked for
liberal candidates whenever I could. I had black friends, and I read
the *New York Times* a lot more frequently than the Bible. If I came
home with a new cause, my parents nodded politely, and waited until
somebody could change the subject.

"One day, years later, something hit me, a kind of epiphany. If I
was always doing and thinking the opposite of what my parents did
and said, they still defined me. Being the opposite of bad doesn't
make you good. It just makes you the mirror image of bad.

"As I examined my beliefs, which I had always been proud of, I
realized that each one was derived in the same reflexive way: I looked
at people I thought were bad, and I made sure my beliefs didn't match
theirs in any way; I looked at people I thought were good, and I made
sure my beliefs were exactly the same as theirs. Nothing I believed in
was original. If being closed-minded is the same as not thinking for
yourself, that was me."

So what is an open mind? I asked.

"It can't be a set of beliefs, no matter how good you think they
are," said Carla. "Most people hold their beliefs in order to feel good
about themselves, not seeing the trap they're falling into. The most lib-
erating idea eventually turns into a shackle if you don't keep changing."

This example points to the pros and cons of reflection. *Pro:* If
you look honestly at your beliefs and assumptions, you can head off
conditioning before it becomes too deep. Your mind won't get stuck
as easily. You will learn how to be more flexible. Healthy doubt will

keep you from falling into conformity. You open the way to become an original person, not simply a carbon copy of a social type. *Con:* Reflection tends to remain mental. It doesn't move much energy in the body. As a result, its power to erase the imprints of conditioning usually isn't very strong. You wind up seeing what's wrong without going deep enough to create change. Reflection is also slow and time-consuming. It can even work against change by creating uncertainty and hesitancy—a problem begins to seem too complex and shaded. If reflection turns into just another habit, you don't act with any kind of spontaneity. By adulthood, people are supposed to lose the reckless-ness of youth, and learning to reflect on your own actions is a large part of that. On the other hand, I don't think I've met many reflective people who have changed their hidden stuck-energy patterns. They do a better job than average of not falling into thoughtless habits, but when their bodies really need change and not just their assumptions, reflection does them little good.

Contemplation involves holding one thing in the mind and letting it unfold. A religious person may contemplate God's mercy, for example. To do that, he lets his mind roam over the topic, seeing images of mercy, feeling what it's like to be merciful or receive mercy. (You may notice a connection to what I'm calling subtle action. They are alike, but subtle action has a specific intent behind it, while con-templation doesn't—it's more a way of letting go.) If the process is allowed to really open up, a contemplative mind can reach very deep. The main effect is to train your mind not to focus on single, isolated details. That kind of sharp focus almost always leads to a struggle with the thing you want to get rid of, and as we saw, struggle only makes conditioning worse by repeating the same conflict over and over.

Contemplation is a technique that need not be tied to religion or spiritual practices, venerable as that tradition is. You can take any bad habit and contemplate what it's all about, persisting until answers begin to come. Those answers will move your energy in new directions.

Tyrone is a high-energy type who threw himself into online trading in high-risk investments. "By my mid-twenties I envied floor traders on Wall Street, the guys you see on TV, yelling, shoving, and going crazy during big market moves," he says. "I had no chance of moving to New York and breaking into that, but ten years ago the Internet offered everyone a chance to be a gunslinger. I jumped in, and pretty soon every free moment had me glued to the screen.

"I didn't have much money, so I bought on margin, which allowed me to make bigger and bigger bets. My risk-taking got bolder, and right away my wins were bigger than my losses. Before I knew it, my account was in six figures, and the top was nowhere in sight. I felt elated. Every morning I couldn't wait for the markets to open."

"Would you call yourself addicted?" I asked.

Tyrone shook his head. "The thought never crossed my mind. The day came when I was only a few trades away from making a million dollars. That was my benchmark. Once I crossed the million-dollar line, my life would change completely. That's what I told myself."

"But you never did cross it," I said.

"I was a beginner, and I had only experienced success. So when my luck turned sour, I went into shock. I lost all my money, and all the money friends had given me to invest when they learned what a genius I was. I was shattered. Guilt and self-recrimination kept me up at night. Some people commiserated. They told me that trading isn't for everyone; it takes toughness and nerves of steel."

"Which only made you feel more inadequate," I commented. "What happened after that?"

"I got back on my feet, slowly, and with fewer friends. But one friend, who was quite a bit older, told me something important. 'Don't think about the money,' he said. 'Think about what money means to you.' I got into trouble, he said, by not knowing that in the first place.

"I'm not sure why I took his advice, but I sat and really looked at it. Two big things came up right away: I liked the thrill of gambling, so money meant adrenaline; I felt like I wasn't good enough, so money meant self-respect. At first, both those things were all right with me. So what if I like to gamble? Why not earn a little self-respect? If I hadn't been feeling so terrible, I might have let it go at that. But I kept going, and one day I felt in my body exactly what the sensations of being on a gambling high were like. The adrenaline rush was there, my heart pounding and everything, but what I hadn't noticed was my anxiety. What I had been calling a thrill contained a lot of fear, worry, and tension.

"As for self-respect, how could I claim that it had improved? I squirreled myself away in front of a glowing computer screen. My mood yo-yoed up and down with every tick of the market. I felt like a hero when I was winning and a loser when I was down. Don't think it was easy for me to see all this. I was drinking antacids out of the bottle for two months after I crashed. But I let all the bad times flow through me again, and whenever they came back, I'd feel them rather than push them down again. The only way out is through, right? Eventually I was at peace. I could admit that I was an out-of-control gambler, an addict who had ignored everything but his compulsion. I expanded out of that suffocating straitjacket. I started to breathe the same air as normal people."

"Do you consider yourself recovered?" I asked.

He looked thoughtful. "I'm not sure. I'm relieved that I broke my old habit. I don't have a jones for trading anymore. And I'm relieved that I'm not tearing myself up with stress anymore. On the other hand, it's been almost ten years, and I still relive the torture of losing all that money. I've turned my life around, but those impressions take a long, long time to fade."

Tyrone's story points out the pros and cons of contemplation.

On the positive side, contemplation can break the boundaries of narrow thinking. It can uncover hidden issues and allow them enough space so that their distorted energy is released. The process of letting go requires no struggle. You can face your demons at your own pace. If you keep focusing on your weak spots with diligence, they will be healed by an expanded sense of self—you will see yourself as bigger than your problems, and that awareness has a tremendous healing power.

On the downside, letting go isn't reliable. If your mind is confused and conflicted, it may be too restless and easily distracted to focus. Your focus may be too weak to actually move any large amount of stuck energy. Looking closely at your problems can create discouragement and depression. You may hate what you see and give yourself reasons to stop looking.

Speaking personally, I think contemplation is more powerful than reflection. It gets into emotions and sensations, while reflection tends to remain intellectual. Some hands-on healers like to say, "The issues are in the tissues," meaning that you must get to the level in the body where the deepest impressions are lodged. Looking and letting go brings results. On the other hand, I don't know many people who have the patience to return to the same focus day after day without getting bored and worn out.

Meditation involves the search for a level of awareness that isn't conditioned. It takes the mind in its restless, confused state and leads it to a higher state that is clear and steady. This process is known as *transcending*. Countless traditions of meditation originated in India and China before spreading throughout the East, but they have in common the same notion of how reality works. Reality flows from finer to grosser states. First there is silence and stillness, then there are subtle objects of the mind (thoughts, emotions, sensations), and finally there are solid objects and the material world itself. When you meditate, you move back upstream, so to speak, going beyond the material world, then beyond the mind that's full of thoughts, emotions, and sensations, finally to arrive at stillness and silence.

This journey is more than a subjective experience, however. Sitting in silence would be no better than sitting in a whirl of thoughts, if both were merely subjective states. In actuality, you transcend from one level of reality to another. Each level contains different kinds of energy, and as you bring in higher energy, your body adapts. Studies of long-term meditators show that markers for health improve, such as reduced blood pressure and stress hormones. But the body can adapt in far more profound ways.

If you touch the right trigger point in your mind, a long-standing distortion in your energy can instantly disappear. Unlike reflection and contemplation, the purpose of meditation is to find the switch that will turn off the automatic behavior created by your old conditioning. I don't mean that lightning strikes all at once. Meditating is a process; it takes time. But the process can cause a sudden change, the way digging a well goes through layer after layer of dirt until suddenly you hit clear, flowing water. I've met many people to whom this has happened, including a man named David, now well past sixty.

"I grew up loathing my father. The full realization of my hatred came very early, when I was nine. It was Christmas, and I was assigned to find the bad bulb when a string of lights went out. As I unscrewed each bulb to test it, I accidentally slipped my finger in a socket. I got a jolt of electricity that threw me backwards. At the same time, the whole tree lit up for a second because my finger completed the circuit.

"As I lay on the floor in shock, I saw that my father was laughing. The sight of the tree lighting up was comical to him, like something out of a cartoon. At that instant I suddenly understood that he couldn't care less about me. I burst out crying, and my father frowned. 'You're the oldest boy in the family,' he said. 'I expect you to start acting like a man.'

"Decades later I happened to visit a psychic, and she immediately told me that I had this old energy of hatred inside me. She said, 'Visualize your relationship with your father. Don't think about it intellectually. Relax and tell me what image comes to mind.'

"I closed my eyes, and I saw two knights covered from head to foot in armor. They were whacking away at each other with broadswords, relentlessly and brutally, but neither one fell down. They just kept battling on. The psychic said that this was my father and me, and that I'd never get rid of my hatred until I found a way for that image to dissolve."

"Did you take her seriously?" I asked.

David gave a wry smile. "I couldn't get past the feeling that my father was a selfish, heartless bastard. He had hurt every member of my family one way or another. Years went by. Eventually, a girlfriend talked me into meditating. I liked it. After each session I felt more relaxed and quiet inside. Then one day my father called without warning—he was almost seventy at the time—and I noticed that the sound of his voice didn't make me bristle.

"The next day I did my morning meditation, after which I lay on the floor to rest, which is what I had been taught to do. The teacher told me that it's necessary to rest because the mind needs time to absorb the deeper awareness it has been exposed to. Unexpectedly I saw the image of two knights again, still hacking away with their broadswords. This time a small voice asked me if I saw any reason to stop fighting. Only one came to mind: I was getting exhausted. This fight had gotten nowhere. My damn sword was heavy! Believe it or not, that did it."

"What do you mean?" I asked.

"The energy of hatred vanished. Even though I felt totally justified in loathing my father, I let go. Or maybe it let go of me. Within a month I had only the vaguest recollection of my old hatred. Within a year I went back home and actually smiled at him. For the first time since I was a boy, I could be around my father comfortably. Sometimes, to my amazement, I feel real affection for him. I was healed in a way I never expected to be."

David's story points out the pros and cons of meditation.

On the plus side, meditation goes to the source. It takes you away from the level of the problem to the level of the solution, which is stuck energy. It releases you from the obligation to dwell in negative thoughts and fight against bad impulses. It is effortless, silently dissolving old conditioning. The overall effect is general—instead of focusing on one issue at a time, meditation carries the whole mind beyond problems.

There are no innate drawbacks to meditation, but there are pitfalls. The wrong kind of meditation simply doesn't work. It may bring on a hint of transcendence—a temporary sense of peace and calm, passing moments of silence, a settled contentment. If you are depressed, meditation may cause you to dwell too much inside yourself. The same is true for people who are introverted: they may retreat inside without reaching a deeper level of awareness. The test of whether meditation is working comes down to energy: if you aren't moving old, stuck energy, your meditation isn't effective.

The benefits of meditation rest on the ability of awareness to change reality. Now we know why that's valid. The chain of events that ends in the body begins in consciousness. By moving stuck energy, the free flow of consciousness is restored, which is enough to bring the body back into a healthy state. Remember, even though we divide problems into the categories of physical, mental, emotional, and so on, the chain of events is the same. To say that someone like David held his anger at the emotional level would be too limited. He held it at the energy level, and his body had adapted, from the brain with its angry thoughts to the cells in his body that responded to the brain's signals. Between them, awareness and energy are the most powerful healers in existence. With that in mind, here are three simple meditations that can set you on the path of healing:

1. *Meditation on the breath.* Sit quietly with your eyes closed. Gently put your attention on the tip of your nose. Breathe in and out normally, and as you do, feel the air flowing through your nostrils. Envision your breath as a faint cloud of pale golden light going in and out of your nose. Feel the soft energy being carried by your breath. Let it relax you and still your mind, but easily, without forcing anything to happen. The process will take care of itself. To help keep your attention from wandering, you can add the sound "hoo" as you exhale.

2.　*Meditation on the heart.* Sitting quietly with your eyes closed, rest your attention on your heart. You don't need to be anatomically precise. Simply find a place in the center of your chest where your attention can rest easily. As you breathe in and out naturally, keep your attention there. Allow any feelings and sensations to arise and pass. If your attention wanders, gently bring it back to rest on your heart.

3.　*Meditation on the light.* Sitting quietly with your eyes closed, envision a soft mixture of white light tinged with gold flowing through your body. See the light come up from your feet and fill your torso. Watch it continue up through your chest and head until it comes out through the crown of your head and goes straight up until it disappears from view. Now envision the same sparkling light descending back down, first entering through the crown of your head. It reverses the upward path from head to chest to torso, exiting the body through the soles of your feet. Once you have mastered this visualization, time it with your breathing. On the inhale, slowly draw the light up from your feet and out the top of your head. On the exhale, draw the light in through the top of your head and out through your feet. Don't force the rhythm. Breathe slowly and naturally in a relaxed state as you perform the visualization.

In Your Life: A Softer Kind of Awareness

Certain eye exercises can teach people how to relax their vision through "soft focus." Because unhealthy energy is hard, rigid, and stuck, it's helpful to learn how to have "soft awareness." I don't mean a woozy blissfulness, but a state of mind that is open, relaxed, and receptive. In that state, you give yourself the best opportunity to flow with life instead of putting up barriers and resistance.

As regards eyesight, hard focus is specific and particular. You take aim, so to speak, and keep an object in your sights. Soft focus widens the field of vision. Instead of isolating one tree, you see the whole forest. I don't know if this approach will actually improve a person's eyesight, but it is very beneficial when applied to the mind. A tightly focused mind becomes narrow and linear if it can't expand. We are all guilty of following narrow mental grooves, like a train confined to one narrow set of tracks. We experience our minds one thought at a time. What this habit leads us to miss is true understanding, because your mind is much more than one event after another.

It is even more futile to try to control your mind one thought at a time. No matter how many years you spend judging your thoughts—rejecting the ones you dislike, and censoring those of which you disapprove—your mind will keep bringing them around. In fact, bad thoughts are more likely to return, as every guilty person knows.

Soft focus sees the mind as a whole. You view thinking as if on a wide screen, accepting that any possible thought can come along. Instead of being a problem, the endless flow of thought becomes the fertile ground of change. The flood cannot be tamed. Nor should we want it to be, because the glory of the mind is that it draws from a thousand springs. Every mental event is temporary: it exists in the moment and then vanishes. Yet, strangely enough, the present moment is connected to eternity, because the present is the only time that is constantly renewed.

Do you see your mind through soft or hard focus? Let me give you some practical distinctions:

Hard Focus

Your mind is overworked. It's exhausting keeping up with it.
You feel a strong aversion to guilty and shameful thoughts.
You push bad memories down out of sight.

You wish you had more control over your thoughts.

You berate yourself when you make a mistake. You call yourself an idiot or stupid.

You struggle between good and bad impulses.

Images you don't want to see pop up anyway, as if on their own.

A strong voice tells you if you are being good or bad.

You find yourself being vigilant in case something unexpected should happen.

You know God sees you, but you try not to think about that.

As you can see, hard focus stands for more than a habit of mind. It's the quality of attention you are paying to yourself and the world. The act of seeing is never neutral. If your attention is wary, hypervigilant to every kind of risk, worried about what can go wrong, your quality of attention is unhealthy. (I'm reminded of the woman who visited her doctor twice a year, every time suspecting that she had cancer. Her checkups were good for fifty years, but finally the day came when her tests revealed that she did have cancer. "See?" she said self-righteously. "I told you so!" Doctors exchange this story to reinforce the point that patients are stubborn, but I can't help thinking about what kind of life the woman had for fifty years until her worst nightmare finally came true.)

A different quality of attention is developed by soft focus.

Soft Focus

Your mind is calm and not overworked. You enjoy being in its presence.

You don't feel haunted by guilty and shameful thoughts.

Your memories fill out your experience; you accept them for what they are.

You don't try to control your thoughts. The more freely they come, the better.

When you make a mistake, you accept it and quickly move on. Not every idea can be perfect or brilliant, and mistakes are often the best teachers.

There's a contrast between good and bad impulses, but you take both in stride. Sometimes you take secret delight in so-called bad thoughts, knowing that they're just another part of your experience.

Unpleasant mental images don't make you afraid or disgusted. You can adapt to the mind's darker side.

You aren't plagued by a judgmental voice telling you that you're bad or unworthy.

You aren't braced for the next disaster around the corner.

If God is looking down on you, he approves of what he sees.

Each item here translates into a new way of approaching your life. Having looked over this list, you may be surprised at how many aspects of hard focus you have accepted as positive. I hope they don't look that way anymore. Once you see that soft focus is a healthier way to relate to your mind, it's much easier to bring positive change into your life. After all, what you see you can heal; what you don't see will remain the same.

Habits of mind are elusive. At the moment we cannot prove that hard focus directly injures the body while soft focus heals it. But because the body is only energy, and because energy is altered by awareness, the value of having healthy awareness speaks for itself. We attach positive value to things for all kinds of reasons, influenced from birth by parents, friends, school, peer groups, and society in general. For good or ill, these influences narrow the mind by fixing its beliefs and assumptions. If you were brought up in a family environment where rigid distinctions were made between right and wrong, where being judgmental came naturally, and where perfection, discipline, and self-control were preached, any and all of these influences will have become internalized over time. Children have no resistance

to having their minds shaped. At the social level, we are so accus-
tomed to viewing the world in terms of heroes and villains, us-versus-
them, winners and losers, that these harsh divisions become habits of
mind. It takes a conscious shift to move from hard to soft focus, and
yet that is a powerful way to dissolve the energy that glues rigid habits
in place.

Breakthrough #4

You Can Improve Your Genes

A breakthrough sometimes comes from seeing a simple truth hidden behind a tangle of complications. Genes are the most complicated thing about the body. Yet there is a simple truth behind them, which is this: you can change your genes, and therefore you can improve them. You are talking to your genes when you do simple things like eating and moving. That's why a recent study showed that people who alter their lifestyle significantly—by eating better, exercising more, and practicing meditation—caused changes affecting perhaps five hundred genes. The changes supported their new lifestyle, and they started within a few weeks. But we should have suspected all along that genes don't sit in a remote castle as silent observers. Even a strong emotion may be enough to alter a gene, because emotions require a shift in brain chemistry—brain cells secrete new chemicals for sadness or happiness, confidence or shyness, when their genes tell them to. The most seemingly stable part of the body turns out to be amazingly fluid and flexible. The code of life is a streaming message that never ends.

Biologists used to claim—and many people think they still do—that we are born with a set of genes that are fixed and unchangeable. But that's like saying we were born with a pair of hands that are unchangeable. In fact, if you are a concert pianist and you have a twin who became a bricklayer, your two hands would be completely different in appearance, flexibility, and skill. Those differences would be reflected in different brain patterns. Your motor cortex will be imprinted with piano playing, your twin's with bricklaying. Identical twins are born with the same set of genes, yet if you take their genetic profile at age seventy, their genes are totally different.

What has changed is a realization that genes only affect you if they are switched on; they have no effect if they are switched off.

Twins are only born identical; they go through life having unique experiences, and those experiences switch some genes on and others off. Everyone's body is the end product of a lifelong process that turns switches on or off. Along the way, three possibilities can occur:

A gene may turn on and off on a fixed schedule.
A gene may turn on and off depending on the person's behavior and experiences.
A gene may turn on and off as a combination of the above.

Two out of the three possibilities leave room for you to choose what your genes will do. This is good news, because for decades we've been told that genes are fixed. They give us our inherited traits and determine what happens in our bodies. Almost no room was left for choice. Yet you don't have to be a twin to wind up at age seventy with a unique genetic profile—it happens to all of us. You are working with the same three possibilities: your behavior won't affect certain genes, it will have a strong effect on others, and for the vast majority of your genes, nature and nurture both play a crucial role.

When people think about genes, the example of blue eyes always comes to mind. If you have inherited a specific gene, your eyes will be blue, and if you have a different gene, your eyes will be brown, green, or hazel. It turns out that this is the exception, however, not the rule. There is no single gene that determines height, for example. The latest research shows that more than twenty genes are involved in how tall a person will grow (some experts raise the number to one hundred genes), and even when they are analyzed, those genes can't tell you if one baby will grow up to be short and another tall. There is a general correlation that a mother's height influences her son's, and a father's height influences his daughter's, but we all know children who are drastically taller or shorter than their parents. When two short parents give rise to a very tall child, nobody really can explain why. Scientists can't even decide if genes account for 90 percent of height—the old conclusion—or as little as 30 percent.

Outside factors aren't reliable predictors, either. We might assume that a better diet makes people taller, but the younger generation in the Philippines is growing shorter despite better economic conditions. We might assume that a tall ethnic group would keep growing taller, but the Plains Indians were among the tallest people on earth when Europeans settled America, and now they aren't. Americans were taller than their European counterparts throughout the eighteenth and nineteenth centuries, but now the Dutch have surpassed them, along with several Scandinavian nations. The pace of change can be fast or slow. The Dutch took 150 years to become the tallest people in the world; the Japanese have jumped up in height just since World War II. (In the animal kingdom, there were only forty breeds of dogs in the world before a craze for developing new breeds swept through Victorian England. Since 1870, that number has jumped to four hundred.)

A few decades ago, medical researchers found that diabetes and sickle-cell anemia ran in families through inherited genes, and wondered if perhaps the same was true for other traits, like depression and schizophrenia, that also seem to run in families. Hope grew that eventually all disorders, physical and mental, could be detected and cured at the genetic level. Parents could find comfort in the knowledge that their child-rearing skills didn't create mental disturbances in their offspring. People suffering from depression, anxiety, obesity, and a host of other complaints could stop worrying that their choices had created the problem. Genes were at fault, and genes would come to the rescue.

If mapping human DNA was the Holy Grail ten years ago, now there are a thousand holy grails—attributing a specific gene to every specific disorder. News stories flood the media about a so-called fat gene, or a gene for Alzheimer's, and perhaps even a gene that makes people believe in God, the "faith gene." All of these announcements wound up bearing little fruit. The single-gene theory is quickly being abandoned, although the public continues to believe in it. In recent years, moreover, the genomes of thousands of individuals have been mapped, and to the shock of researchers, there turn out to be at least 3 million differences in the genetic makeup of any two people (a huge number considering that we possess only 20,000 to 30,000 genes, far less than anyone supposed).

Genes cannot govern all the other factors that make you who you are. A gene didn't give you a love for gardening, a mania for collecting postage stamps, a taste for Bach, or an image of the person you would fall in love with. What would happen, though, if we stopped looking at DNA physically? Let's bring genes into the field of awareness and see how they respond. DNA is a memory bank storing every experience from the past that makes us human. Instead of letting those memories use you, you can learn to use them.

Your DNA is no more physical than other parts of your body; it is made of energy, and you can change its energy patterns through a change of awareness. You were born with some predispositions that will determine how your body turns out, yet as you inject your own desires, habits, and intentions, a fixed trait will turn out to be very malleable—a mere wisp of desire is enough to affect DNA. How ironic that the two things that medicine thought were fixed, the brain and DNA, turn out to be the keys for reinventing the body.

Mariel's story

The big question isn't whether you can improve your genes, but how far you can take the process. Genes stand in the way of change only because we accept that they have power over us. Yet some people find a way to overcome their genes. Mariel, now in her thirties, was born with a congenital eye defect that couldn't be corrected with surgery. "I grew up knowing that my sight would fade away as I grew older," she said. "As the years went by, I faced the challenge of constantly adjusting to new limitations. By the time I was out of college and going to graduate school, small print was very hard to read."

One day Mariel was in the library and found herself unable to read the card catalog. "They had just switched to a microfiche system, and trying to make out the tiny print on the screen was very frustrating. On an impulse, I got up and walked into the stacks. I headed to the general area where the book I wanted was located. When I got there, I intended to ask for help, but since no one was around, I reached up at random and grabbed a volume. It turned out to be the very one I wanted."

At the time Mariel saw this as a coincidence, albeit an extraordinary one. But over time a pattern began to emerge. "I found that I could see without using my eyes. I was able to recover lost objects like keys or a wallet without having to search high and low. At first I assumed that I was just retracing my steps, the way most people do when they lose something. But one day I came home from a restaurant to find that my checkbook was gone. Before I could even try to recall where I left it, a visual image flashed in my mind, showing a checkbook lying in a very specific place in the restaurant parking lot. It had fallen out of my purse when I pulled out my car keys. So I went back to the retaurant, and the checkbook was lying exactly where I'd envisioned it."

Mariel came to rely on her newfound second sight. "If I'm writing a paper and need a specific citation, all I need to do is open the reference book and the pages will fall open to the passage I want. This doesn't happen every single time, but it seems to work just when I need it most."

"What's your explanation for this?" I asked.

"It was tempting to think there was a special connection between me and God," she said. "Then I ran across an article by a neurologist about sighted people who suddenly become blind, usually in an accident. Some people simply resign themselves to being sightless, but others adapt in amazing ways. One blind man took up roofing. He specialized in extremely complex roofs with multiple gables and steep pitches. He preferred working at night, much to the consternation of the neighbors. These were roofs that even a sighted person would be wary of climbing on in full daylight. Another person I recall developed a skill for designing intricate gearboxes whose complex workings he saw only in his mind's eye. He hadn't had this skill before a sudden leak of acid sprayed him in the eyes and blinded him. Only then did he discover that he possessed this remarkable ability."

Everyone's genes hide secret potential. One need only turn to the work of the late Dr. Paul Bach-y-Rita from Mexico, who attracted general scorn thirty years ago when he suggested that the brain was capable of "sensory substitution." That is, a blind person could learn to "see," for example, by substituting the sense of touch for the sense of sight. Braille already gave us a clue that something akin to this audacious idea was possible, but Dr. Bach-y-Rita went much further. By the time of his death at age seventy-two, he had developed a mechanism known as a "Brain Port," a small paddle that fits on the tongue. Using a grid of six hundred electrical points attached to a camera, the Brain Port can deliver a picture to the tongue of whatever the camera sees. This picture consists of electrical impulses conducted to sensory receptors for touch, yet after some practice, the blind person's brain actually "sees" the image.

The evidence is not just anecdotal. MRIs have shown that the visual cortex of a blind person lights up when signals are sent to the tongue. In a recent report on public television, one could watch blind patients throwing a tennis ball into a trash can from twenty feet and walking a curving path without going out of bounds. But sensory substitution goes further. A woman who had lost her sense of balance as a side effect of an antibiotic could not be helped by drugs or surgery because the entire vestibular labyrinth in her inner ear had been rendered completely useless. Yet by training with the Brain Port, which told her tongue when she was upright and when she wasn't, she regained her balance. Something even more remarkable followed. When the woman took off the Brain Port device that enabled her to balance herself, she didn't immediately lose her balance again. One hour of training held good for about an hour after it ended. As she progressed, a day of training held good for a day afterward. Eventually, to the amazement of the experimenters, she could walk and ride a bicycle without wearing the Brain Port device at all.

The brain's vestibular system is extremely complex, and yet much or all of it found a substitute elsewhere, in a region of the brain that formerly wasn't devoted to equilibrium at all. Not only has Dr. Bach-y-Rita proved his point that the brain is more flexible than commonly supposed, but his research suggests that the brain is much more creative as well. How does an organ that is mostly water, governed entirely by electrochemical impulses, know that a person needs a new way of sensing, one that so far as we know isn't necessary to human evolution?

Seeds of change

The brain's hidden potential comes down to the gene's hidden potential. A brain cell can't make a new move unless its DNA sends out new chemical signals. Instead of getting tangled up in organic chemistry, which will never transcend the physical level anyway, you need to realize that you are talking to your genes all the time. For every trait that is fixed, such as eye, hair, and skin color, myriad genes are weaving a complex pattern of response to the following factors:

How you think.
How you feel.
How you act.
What you believe.
What you expect.
The threats you fear.
The objects of your desires.
The lifestyle decisions you make.
The relationships you focus on.
Your immediate environment.
Your habits and preferences.

At the most basic level, lifestyle choices have genetic consequences. In the wellness movement, approaches such as vegetarian diets, Hatha Yoga, meditation, and psychosocial support have long been seen as good preventive measures. Now it seems that adopting these approaches may stop or even reverse serious illness—heart disease, diabetes, high blood pressure, prostate cancer, obesity, high cholesterol, and other chronic conditions show promising signs in this area. Only recently has research gone to the genetic level of explaining these beneficial changes. Hundreds of genes, it has been found, may be changing their expression in as little as a few months after patients change their lifestyle in a positive direction. Genes associated with cancer, heart disease, and inflammation were down-regulated or "turned off," whereas protective genes were up-regulated or "turned on."

At this moment you are making all kinds of choices that weave together the quirky, unpredictable, and creative patterns of your life. Do your genes care? As it happens, they do, very much. It's been shown that death rates rise significantly after Christmas, for example, and the same spike occurs after mortally ill people have a birthday. The implication is that when someone is dying, she can postpone her time of death until after a day she wants to live to see. (I know of a man slowly dying from brain cancer who passed away when a Lakota Sioux medicine man was brought into his sickroom and performed a ceremony to release the spirit from the body so that it could reach the afterlife.)

It's as if having a desire is enough to tell your body what to do. Is that enough with genes as well? Influencing a gene used to be considered impossible, but the situation is rapidly changing. Genetic researchers working with mice found that baby mice that were well mothered turned into healthier specimens than baby mice who were badly mothered. A mouse who's a good mother licks and cleans her offspring almost all the time and stays physically close to them. A bad mouse mother is erratic about grooming her offspring, and wanders away from them. As a result, her offspring grow up to be more susceptible to stress. They are more easily frightened and also show less curiosity about the world, and less willingness to explore it.

In itself, this finding wasn't dramatic. It had been shown long ago that baby monkeys who were not allowed to cling to their mothers and be nurtured by them grew up emotionally disturbed (you may remember the poignant photos of forlorn infant rhesus monkeys clinging to a wire-mesh imitation of a mother monkey). The radical part of the mouse experiment came when it was discovered that mice who experienced bad mothering turned into bad mothers themselves. They neglected to groom their own offspring enough, and tended to wander away. In other words, the baby mice of bad mothers didn't acquire new genes, yet they did acquire a new behavior. Suddenly that first early human who decided to stand upright to view the far horizon may not be tied to genes. He may have passed on his new behavior to his children without waiting millennia for a new mutation. But how?

The answer lies at an obscure cellular level known as *epigenes*. Every strand of DNA is wrapped in a buffer of complex proteins—the epigene—that somehow trigger a gene to turn on or off. When the epigene is affected by something you do or feel, it won't create new DNA—your genetic inheritance remains the same as at birth. But its behavior can change drastically. So, when a bad mouse mother warps the normal development of her baby, what matters is that the baby's DNA is activated to start behaving badly, eventually passing on the same bad behavior to future generations. I've given a negative example, yet many positive implications open up if we can learn to switch genes on and off. Gene therapy has been a failure in treating cancer, for example, but epigenes may come to the rescue. Because gene therapy tries to replace or change the genes you were born with, the body rebels, producing many undesirable side effects. On the other hand, if the epigene can tell your DNA to prevent a tumor from growing, or to stop the tumor after it starts, then cancer could be defeated simply by asking a cell to behave differently.

If switching a gene on and off is the most natural way to create change, how do we gain control over the switch? Lifestyle changes are a start, but perhaps we possess more direct control, only the switch is hidden. To stay with cancer, there are thousands of documented cases in which an advanced malignancy has disappeared without treatment. These spontaneous remissions, as they are known, have created a vast mythology. All it takes is a rumor that some herb, fruit concoction, gem or color therapy, religious ritual, prayer, or miraculous intervention has saved a life, and dying cancer patients will desperately pursue that avenue. Nobel Prize winner Linus Pauling was convinced that megadoses of vitamin C had cured a small group of terminally ill cancer patients. Complete blood transfusions and so-called blood purification are offered illicitly in Mexico. Because they are labeled as alternative treatments, a vast array of therapies exist whose actions remain completely unknown and unproven.

What we do know is that in rare cases an *x* factor can cause tumors to retreat for no known reason. It can even happen without any treatment at all: a certainty simply dawns on some patients that they will recover, and their certainty is borne out. That is more in line with traditional faith healing, which attributes cures to an invisible higher power and nothing physical at all. What may unite these wildly disparate approaches (after weeding out the frauds and false rumors) is the power of awareness to switch on a tumor-suppressing gene.

We find ourselves caught in a dilemma. Hope that brings results can't be called false. On the other hand, reducing all alternative therapies to hope-mongering would be unfair. There may be an unpredictable combination of substance and spirit at work, where a patient's subjective hope and belief enables a therapy to work. The challenge is very basic: How do you effectively take control of your genes?

Tuning in, tuning out

All of us cause changes to our genes, but it's a special skill to do so consciously. We aren't tuned in to the level of our bodies that actively switches genes on and off. It turns out, however, that this level of awareness is available. You can't go there to target one gene directly, but there's no need to. You only need to tune in. Tuning your body out is the single greatest harm you can do. Without a clear channel of communication, you can't expect your cells to respond to your desires and intentions. "Tuning out" is shorthand for withdrawing your attention, judging against your body, and ignoring its signals. As with everything else, there are different degrees of tuning out. Depending on how disconnected you become, your body will send back increasingly severe reactions: *absence of pleasure, reduced vitality, discomfort, numbness,* and *pain.*

Progressing from one stage to another can take years, but a sudden trauma like a car accident or serious illness can decrease body awareness quickly and dramatically. When someone near to us dies and we go into grief, for example, the whole spectrum is there: food no longer tastes good (absence of pleasure); we feel listless and tired (reduced vitality); the body feels heavy and sleep doesn't come easily (discomfort); sensations like heat and cold aren't felt, and familiar surroundings seem alien and strange (numbness); random aches in the body come and go (pain). There are always mental consequences as well, and quite often people who feel depressed, numb, and empty inside don't realize that they are seriously disconnected from their bodies.

Here's a list of what it typically feels like to tune out. Read the list over and ask yourself how many items apply to you personally.

You feel detached from your body and what it's saying.

You find it hard to feel physical pleasure.

You compare your body unfavorably to that of other people, or to some ideal of the "perfect" body.

You feel ugly or unworthy in the body you have.

It makes you unhappy to imagine your body shape.

Being touched makes you uncomfortable.

You tend to misinterpret other people's physical approach as aggressive or, at the very least, startling.

Bonding through physical intimacy isn't an option.
You feel clumsy and uncoordinated.
The only time you liked your body was when you were young.
You physically don't consider yourself feminine enough, or masculine enough.
Your body sometimes doesn't seem to belong to you.

These negative attitudes range from mild to severe. Yet your body always senses when it is being ignored or judged unfavorably. For most people, ignoring their bodies has become a habit. Exposing their bodies to undue stress scarcely brings a second thought. After all, don't we assume that modern life has turned stressful, beyond our individual control? If you were really tuned in to your body, you'd feel its discomforts before they demanded your attention. Tuning in comes down to becoming more aware. The more aware you are, the more sensitive you are to your body, and vice versa.

Seen symbolically, all disorders are cases where the body becomes a stranger, an enemy, a failed ally, or a defeated victim. To prevent those metaphors from turning into reality, you need to offer reassurance to your body that you will care for it, that you will listen when it speaks.

In Your Life: Tuning In

Once you tune in, your body has an amazing capacity to correct itself. To begin this process, you need to feel comfortable in your body. There has to be a basic connection that isn't blocked by guilt, shame, and discomfort. If you take the following quiz, it will show you where the work of reconnecting starts for you personally.

Are You at Home in Your Body?

The list below covers the most common things that people feel uncomfortable with when it comes to their bodies. Mark your comfort level with each item, as follows:

E - Enjoyable
D - Don't mind
U - Uncomfortable
T - Totally avoid

___ wearing a revealing bathing suit

___ wearing clothes that fit

___ looking in a full-length mirror

___ trying on clothes in a store

___ dancing

___ playing team sports

___ hugging

___ snuggling

___ sex with the lights on

___ being looked at in public

___ describing how you look physically

___ being physically flirtatious

___ thinking about your weight

___ being casually touched by a friend or acquaintance

___ hearing others refer to you physically

___ sitting quietly, particularly in public

___ attempting physical challenges (hiking, running, climbing flights of stairs, etc.)

___ being seen nude by your spouse or lover

___ undressing at the gym

___ having your picture taken

___ thinking about being touched physically

___ buying a bra or other intimate apparel

This isn't a quiz where you tally up your scores; it's a worksheet for getting back in touch with your body. Pick an item that you marked "Uncomfortable," and write a plan for overcoming it. Your plan begins in awareness. Imagine yourself in the uncomfortable situation. Use a specific image that evokes your discomfort so that you feel it emotionally, and possibly even physically.

Be with that energy. Simply by tuning in to it you are taking the first step toward a new body awareness. Don't freeze up or get tense. Breathe easily; relax your body. If the image has to do with undressing at the gym, see yourself standing there, but instead of feeling all eyes on you, create a change. Have people look away and pay no attention. Repeat this new scenario several times. See them staring at you, making you embarrassed, then have them turn away. As you repeat the process, your energy around this issue will start to dissipate.

Now proceed to another aspect of the scene, such as stripping down until you are naked. Use the same process as before. See yourself in your discomfort, and then change the scenario. This time make yourself indifferent to being naked. Maybe you are chatting with a friend or rubbing lotion on your leg. Maybe someone walks by without noticing you. Maybe someone comes up to you as you are taking off your clothes and asks for help with something. The point is to add comfort and ease to the troubling situation. Again, repeat the change, like running a movie scene several times.

The ultimate point of this exercise is to get your awareness to shift, allowing a clearer channel of communication with the body. If you are deeply disconnected from your body, this exercise may be too intimidating. If it is, then instead of beginning with an item marked "Uncomfortable," begin with one marked "Don't mind." Eventually, you will be able to get through all the steps of tuning in:

1. Freeing up stuck energy through visualization.
2. Stepping into the situation you once felt uncomfortable with.
3. Feeling indifferent in the situation, to the point that you don't mind it.

4. Feeling completely comfortable.
5. Enjoying and seeking out the once-avoided situation.

You won't be tuned in until you reach the end of the process. Just keep reminding yourself that every stage of healing takes place in awareness. You won't do yourself any good by abruptly buying a bikini or letting someone touch you intimately before you are mentally and emotionally comfortable. Keep checking in with the sensations brought up by your body. Be with them; look at them. If you keep returning in small visits to your discomfort zone, your body will begin to respond. Trust it, and don't push yourself too hard, too fast.

In addition, expose yourself to the comforts of physical sensations that you've ignored. Look over the times you marked "Enjoy," and give your body the nourishment of positive sensations. Remind yourself that your body is the junction between the visible and invisible worlds. The most pleasurable experiences—of love, warmth, beauty, bonding, and nurturing—bridge those worlds. They have a component that your body understands and a component that your mind understands. Let the two merge into one. Then the process of tuning in is complete.

Breakthrough #5

Time Isn't Your Enemy

When a breakthrough is powerful enough, it can overturn the natural order of things. The whole issue of time fits into this category. Is anything more powerful than time? It rules the cycle of birth and death. It moves forward inexorably. It brings aging and decay. The ultimate liberation for your body would be to overcome the effects of time. In so doing, you would overcome the body's greatest flaw, which is that it breaks down for no better reason, apparently, than the negative effects of the passage of time.

In this breakthrough you will see that time isn't your enemy. We can choose to stop giving in to time as if it ruled our lives. There are signs that this is happening already. The present generation invented the "new old age," which is constantly pushing the biological envelope. In 2005, a Romanian woman named Adriana Illescu became, at age sixty-seven, the oldest mother on record, using in-vitro fertilization to give birth to a healthy baby girl. The event created uneasy feelings around the world, but Illescu's attitude is typical of rapidly changing beliefs.

"I am only sorry that I don't look like a young woman for my daughter," she said. "I am always amazed when I look in the mirror and see myself. There's such a difference between what I feel and what I see."

Illescu has shattered the stereotype of motherhood belonging only to the young by asking her body to keep up with how young she felt, and in doing so she was quite consciously pushing the boundaries of aging.

"A little sports, a little activity, and an active intellectual life lead the body to become younger because there are hormones generated in the brain that make you feel better," she told reporters.

To set a new agenda for the body, attitudes must shift. In the past, old age was feared, and rightly so, because senior citizens were put on the shelf. When attitudes shifted, thanks to better health, longer life spans, and shifting demographics, people began to expect to be vigorous, alert, and useful well beyond the age of sixty-five. A recent poll revealed that more than half of Americans consider seventy to be late middle age and that old age itself didn't begin until after eighty. The oldest man to finish the London marathon is now 101, continuing to show us what is possible for anyone.

And yet slowing down the aging process isn't the same as solving the problem of time. Why do we accept the ravages of time at all? Can the body's worst enemy turn into an ally?

Evolution or erosion?

The problem of time comes down to one thing: your body evolves and erodes simultaneously. Both are constant, invisible forces. The surest way to escape time's clutches is to keep evolving, and the good news is that sometimes evolution gains the upper hand. Then we feel expansive, optimistic, forward-looking, and eager to discover new things. In that mode, we have all the time in the world. We can forget time and live as if it didn't exist (as lovers do, or people totally absorbed in work or play). At other times entropy becomes dominant. Now we don't have time to get important things done, and what time there is wears us down. Bored or depressed, we find our lives losing momentum. As our bodies balance evolution and entropy, the two faces of time silently battle for supremacy. The "new old age" proves that erosion can be resisted through beliefs and attitudes. There is no need to buy into any belief that promotes entropy. Far better to assume, as we have all along, that awareness can change any energy pattern at will.

Familiar as they seem, both of these forces are mysterious. Despite the acceptance of Darwinian evolution by the scientific community, nobody knows why or how Nature takes sudden creative leaps. You would never guess, looking at the fossils of the tiniest dinosaurs that scrambled underfoot as their huge kin shook the earth, that these would be the ultimate survivors of the disaster that wiped huge dinosaurs out. Still less would you have been able to see in their scaly skins the potential for hair, fur, and feathers. But without that hidden possibility, mammals and birds could not have evolved.

Evolution doesn't telegraph what its next creative leap will be. This is especially true in human beings. Our Stone Age ancestors had no skill at mathematics (it is disputed whether Neanderthal man could count; certain Australian aborigines still use a system of "one, two, and many" as their only arithmetic), and yet, hidden in their cerebral cortex was a staggering capacity for advanced calculations. And ordinary memory, which seems quite limited, can expand at will. With practice, you or I could memorize every word of the Bible, and a precious few individuals are gifted with total photographic memory, being able to recall every moment of their lives.

There is no indication that memory has any evolutionary limits, either. It could keep unfolding, without end. The human brain seems set up for that already. A dramatic instance is a woman in her mid-thirties named Jill Price who developed total recall more or less overnight at age fourteen. She describes how one side of her mind participates in everyday reality while the other projects a detailed movie of any day she wants to recall. Not only does she remember what she did on that day, as well as the food served on the family table and the news stories in the daily paper, if Price hears a few bars of a television theme song, she instantly knows the show in question *and the day she heard the theme*. She can name themes from series that were canceled after a handful of episodes.

This extremely rare gift is also a unique burden. Price's memories come with all the original emotions attached. Somewhat overweight, she ruefully remembers every time her mother criticized her appearance. The title of her autobiography is tellingly poignant: *The Woman Who Can't Forget*. Price's onset of total recall was out of her control, but she reminds us of the vastness of human potential. (If every young child was given memory training, would we develop into a society with total recall?)

Entropy looks less mysterious, at least on the surface. It is simply Nature's tendency to disperse energy and become less organized over time. Hot food grows cold if you let it stand; the entire universe grows colder by expanding in all directions, diffusing the original heat generated by the Big Bang. But life stands in opposition to this seemingly inflexible principle: all living things build up energy and become more and more complex. So why wasn't Nature simply satisfied with cooling down? There was no real need for the primordial universe to build DNA, which traps billions of bits of energy along its double helix and gains more energy as we eat and digest food.

Life represents a cosmic capacity to manipulate both time and energy. As long as you take in more energy than you give off, you are stopping time. Time only runs out when energy runs out. Imagine a log in the fireplace that takes an hour to burn. That hour represents how much energy is available before "heat death" occurs. DNA makes energy available forever—or close enough, at two billion years so far, and counting. DNA functions as if it were immortal. Entropy isn't banished; it still presses on your genes, coaxing them to break down, but life persists anyway and keeps evolving. To a physicist, your body is an island of "negative entropy," because as long as it's alive it refuses to cool down. A cell deprived of food and air for as little as three seconds begins to deteriorate; a brain deprived of oxygen for more than ten minutes begins to die. But these aren't threats so long as your body knows how to manage time.

Now that you know the stakes, a choice must be made—evolve or decline—because the option of standing still isn't available. If you sit in a chair and stop using your muscles, they will atrophy; the same holds true if you stop using your brain. The obvious choice is to side with evolution, because then you can grow in new, unexpected areas, giving your body an agenda that time cannot undo.

Controlling time

Mastery over time is built into you. Your body runs on multiple clocks, each set to a different speed. When you were a baby, your skull bones fused at a rate that was incredibly slow compared with the firestorm of new connections that your brain was creating by the millions every minute. Your mother's immune cells, which were your only protection from disease when you were born, were dying as you developed your own antibodies. Your sexual organs were essentially dormant; your adult teeth were the tiniest of seeds. Dozens of different cycles were being controlled by the DNA that was originally contained in one cell, that first fertilized egg. You didn't develop fast DNA for your brain and slow DNA for your skull bones. The same genetic code somehow coordinates events lasting from a few thousandths of a second (the firing of a neuron, the absorption of oxygen by a red blood cell) to a few years (losing your baby teeth, developing a full immune system), to entire decades (mature reasoning, gray hair, menopause).

What this amounts to is that your body is far from being time's victim; on the contrary, it orchestrates time to your benefit. Once you force upon the body your own fears and negative beliefs about time, however, the trouble begins. Take the simple belief that there is never enough time. It's this belief that creates deadlines, a highly symbolic word with overtones of mortality: if you run out of time before you cross the line, you're dead. Your body plays its part in this belief. If you find yourself racing to meet a deadline, your heart rate will speed up, your blood vessels will constrict, and your mind will race to keep pace with everything you need to do. These are all disruptions of bodily rhythms and therefore disruptions of your body's exquisite control of time. What's more damaging is that you are treating time as an adversary.

There are many other ways in which this happens. As we've seen, research on stress has found that one of the biggest causes is uncertainty. If you place a mouse on a metal plate and give it harmless electric shocks at regular intervals, the mouse won't be happy, but it will eventually adjust. If the same harmless shocks are administered at random intervals, however, the mouse grows exhausted to the point of death in a matter of a few days. Since life is full of unpredictability, adapting to it is a major challenge.

It's the incidentals, ironically, that break your body down at the level where time is being controlled. When you focus anti-aging on the physical level—on exercise, diet, vitamins, antioxidants, weight loss, cosmetics, and plastic surgery—you bypass the invisible level that is far more important. Whatever breaks down your body's timing creates aging. The culprit is not time itself. Look at the invisible factors that do the greatest damage:

Unpredictability. Random events disrupt your body's rhythms.
Disorder, confusion. A breakdown of external order leads to inner disorder.
Accidents. Mistakes in your life lead to mistakes in your body.
Trauma, sickness. When wounded, your body loses track of time.
Violence. When attacked, your body's timing is shattered.
Chaos. When all sense of order is destroyed, your body cannot manage time at all.

I've listed these damaging factors from least to most harmful because that's how your body deals with them. It can adapt to unpredictability more easily than to disorder, and to disorder more easily than to accidents. Consider how everyday choices influence your body's timing.

Unpredictability. Choosing to keep irregular hours, working the night shift, going to sleep at different times, eating irregularly, drastically changing how much you eat: all these choices are known to throw off the body's basic metabolic rhythms. The rhythms of the body need to be healthy, because they are the most basic way that you keep your life properly timed—every cell synchronized with every other. The more irregular your lifestyle, the harder it is for this delicate, complex coordination to exist. Correction requires going back to regular hours of work, eating, and sleep. In most cases this is enough to allow the body to reset itself.

Disorder, confusion. Choosing to procrastinate, doubting, indecision, lack of organization, impulsiveness, slovenliness or careless hygiene, lack of purpose, restlessness, drifting: these factors all create a state of external disorder that the body must cope with. The brain

sends confusing signals about what to do, so the cells lack clear direction. The inner and outer are always linked, and bringing order to
your outer life has a beneficial influence on your inner life. The same
is true in reverse: If you address inner confusion and disorder, you can
begin to find ways to put your external affairs in order as well.

Accidents. Choosing to be inattentive, distracted, undisciplined,
unfocused, self-destructive: although some accidents are beyond our
control, most result from a failure to pay attention, which is a choice.
Your cells are in the habit of never forgetting; they must function precisely, thousands of times per second. If your attention to external
things wanders and becomes unfocused, the brain can't be expected to
keep your body in perfect working order, either.

Trauma, sickness. Choosing unnecessary risks and dangers, gambling
with your safety, exposing your body to physical threat and infection,
refusing to pay attention to healing: the belief that sickness strikes
randomly no longer holds true. You open your body to trauma and
disease by ignoring well-known guidelines for healthy living and prevention. At a more subtle level, your immune system takes its cues
from the brain, which implies a great deal of control over when you get
sick and when you don't. Once a serious trauma occurs, that part of
the body can no longer coordinate its activities with the rest of the
body. The loss of one component throws off timing everywhere until
healing brings the whole system back into line.

Violence. Choosing to be out of control, unleashing anger and rage,
refusing to understand your hidden hostility, seeking revenge,
dwelling on resentment. Any eruption of violence calls for an extreme
reaction from your body, firing up every cell to high alert. Adrenaline and other hormones involved in fighting are released; these are
catabolic, meaning that they break down tissue in order to release
energy. As this breakdown occurs on the physical level, control over
time also breaks down—the sudden intrusion of alarm cuts off

normal communications. Emergencies are enormously disruptive in external life, and your inner life mirrors that disruption.

Chaos. Living in the total disorder of war, crime, domestic violence, abandoning all coping mechanisms, going over the edge socially or mentally: at its most extreme, life turns chaotic, and the disasters of outer life are visited on the body. When you can no longer cope, your brain becomes drastically disorganized. The signals sent to the body are then so disordered that the most basic processes of sleep, digestion, metabolism, and healing become seriously compromised. Short bursts of chaos are almost as destructive as living with chaos permanently. In both cases the body runs the risk of becoming so imbalanced that it cannot return to normal functioning on its own.

Fortunately, the order in which the body gets damaged holds true in reverse. You can make choices that prevent erosion. In other words, you can retune your body so that it regains its complex mastery over time. By starting with the easiest step, you lay a foundation, and then it becomes more viable to make difficult choices.

Making Time Your Ally

Keep regular hours, eat and sleep on a regular schedule.

Avoid drastic changes in diet and activity.

Set up an orderly work environment. Reduce distractions.

Rest quietly once to twice during the day to let your body retune itself.

Take yourself out of stressful situations sooner rather than later.

Take your time; don't rush.

Make decisions when they arise. Don't procrastinate or get distracted.

Pay attention to what is directly in front of you. Focus on one thing at a time.

Don't multitask. Dividing your attention leads to confusion and weakened focus.

Avoid the temptation to plunge into high-risk situations.

Stay within your comfort zone.

Put your house and finances in order.

Address underlying anxiety.

Release your repressed anger. Learn to do this without losing control or hurting others.

Renounce violence in thought and word.

Become more resilient emotionally.

Eliminate chaotic influences at work and in your primary relationship.

Live as if you have all the time in the world.

Your ultimate goal, living as if you have all the time in the world, is functional immortality. This happens to be how every cell in your body is already living. Immortality comes naturally; giving in to time is what requires effort. I'm reminded of a therapist I know whose patients' lives seem out of control. He surprises them by saying, "Go home and clean your house. Make your bed every morning. Don't skip breakfast for a week. Get to work fifteen minutes early. Then come back and we'll discuss what's bothering you." He wants to see if they are capable of addressing the simple things that clutter our awareness before turning to deeper psychological issues. Even what looks like a small change can retune the body. That's why we work up to the most damaging things—trauma, violence, and chaos—by starting with the easiest.

If your body can run on dozens of clocks at the same time, each kept in perfect sync, this raises the question of where the master timekeeper resides. It implies that there is a place that is unaffected by time, like sitting on the solid riverbank to watch the constantly changing motion of a river. This place must be outside time, which means that in some way your body knows what it means to be timeless. Functional immortality was born here, in the awareness that time cannot touch us.

Andrea's story

Because your body is timeless at some level, you should be able to experience that. It's a mistake to believe that only a handful of mystics, those deeply devoted to finding God, will experience the timeless. In fact, experiencing the timeless happens spontaneously to all kinds of people, usually when they least expect it. In the middle of life's activity, they suddenly step out of ordinary time. This happened to Andrea, a woman now in her thirties, when she was a grad student in San Francisco.

"I lived on a fellowship that was running out, and then unexpectedly I got pregnant. My boyfriend was totally unsupportive; he was already staggering between part-time jobs trying to finish his Ph.D. thesis. I was twenty-six, and it felt like my whole future was unraveling," Andrea recalls.

"My parents have strict moral views, so I was completely alone when I terminated the pregnancy. The whole procedure was very clinical and nonjudgmental, but I went home in tears. I was so shattered that all I could do was lie down in the bedroom with the blinds down. I was experiencing what they call racing anxiety—my mind whirled with images of all the horrible ways my life could go wrong.

"I must have fallen asleep, because when I woke up I smelled the scent of lemon geraniums. I was a bit groggy, but I knew that scent. I'd bought a tiny lemon geranium at the grocery and stuck it on the windowsill in the kitchen. How could I smell it all the way in the bedroom, with the door closed? Before I could answer, a kind of peace entered me, as if carried by the scent, and a voice on the edge of my awareness asked me to be quiet. At that moment my mind went silent. There were no more thoughts, just dead quiet inside."

"Is silence really dead?" I asked. "Something keeps happening, doesn't it?"

Andrea agreed. "'Dead' is the wrong word. It was a vibrant silence, if that makes any sense. It almost sparkled. After a few moments the vibrancy went away, and nothing was left except a deeper stillness. I felt incredibly safe and supported, if that's the right word, as if I had landed on the ground floor of the mind. Outside the window I heard some children walk by, laughing at something or other. Instantly I merged with the sound. It was uncanny, but their laughter stopped being outside my head—it came from inside me. There was no separation; I also felt bathed by the children's innocence and carefree mood. This feeling lasted for only a minute before they were out of earshot, but it became the turning point in my life."

"In what way?" I asked.

"In every way, I think," said Andrea. "I wasn't the same anymore. I had gone somewhere I didn't know you could go. I've heard of people who have near-death experiences, and when they come back, they're no longer afraid of dying. Sometimes they aren't afraid of anything. I experienced that same shift."

"But you didn't die," I pointed out.

"True," said Andrea. "But think about how sacred silence and stillness are in every culture. 'Be still, and know that I am God,' says the Bible. I don't know if I contacted God, but there was something indescribable in my experience. It was like losing all boundaries, but instead of falling apart, you feel more real. My life didn't become smooth sailing from that day on. I'm not saying that. Yet the outer world doesn't crowd in on me as much as it used to. Even now, years later, I can go back and touch the peace that comes when you know you're a part of everything, and everything is part of you."

When such a moment arrives, it feels like we've stepped outside of time. But how can that be? The basic answer is that we all step outside time on a regular basis. The atoms that make up our bodies wink in and out of the physical universe thousands of times a second. Sometimes a particle that disappears in one place instantaneously reappears in another. Or it sends a signal to another particle light-years away (it can tell the second particle in what direction to spin, for example), and the message crosses billions of miles in an instant, beyond the speed of light.

Strange as that behavior may sound, these are the particles that make up your body, which means that a fundamental aspect of you is quite familiar with the timeless. To make this less exotic, imagine the color red. Once you see the color in your mind's eye, ask a simple question: Where is this red? There are no brain cells that turn red when you think of the color, nor do you go to a special place on earth, a color bank, where red is stored. Redness (or any other hue) exists in a mysterious location that seems to be outside ordinary space and time. You can fetch a color instantaneously whenever you want to see it in your mind's eye, because there was no distance to cover and no time needed to make the journey. The same holds true for how billions of cells manage to be coordinated in your body. There is no master clock ticking away anywhere in your brain—we know this because the brain manages hundreds of different rhythms meshed together. The brain tunes in to a place that's on the very edge of the timeless. By being anchored there, where atoms first begin to vibrate, setting the timing of the entire universe, your brain has found the only place from which time can be managed. Strange as this concept may seem to the rational mind, which depends on clock time to get through the day, the timeless is a familiar place to your cells. They function as if they were immortal, simply because they make use of the timeless every second. The challenge for us is to adopt functional immortality as our basic way of life. To do that, we must reawaken the connection between time and the timeless, which is known as the soul.

In Your Life: Back in the Flow

Once you can accept that time was never your enemy, then escaping the ravages of time becomes possible. It's your mind that started the trouble; it's your body that will get you out of trouble. The mind cuts life up into neat slices—days, weeks, months, years—hoping to hoard as many as possible, but always dreading the end that will inevitably come. By contrast, your body lives in the moment, and each moment merges into another in one continuous flow.

The breakdown of flow is your real enemy. When flow breaks down, the following happens: energy is wasted, communication within the body is cut off, gaps appear in the body's intelligence. These are invisible events, but they are real. Once you learn to restore the flow, however, your body is fully capable of repairing the damage that has built up. It will naturally return to a state of dynamic balance. At that point the whole aging process comes to an end.

No one can expect to bring aging to a stop immediately. But you can make a major difference starting now. Your aim is to align your mind with a new way of being. We've seen the importance of meditation in this regard. Meditation exposes your brain to a less active state, and through repeated exposure, your brain adapts to that stillness and silence. However, there's still the problem of everyday life, which pulls us into our old belief that time is running out. If you want to have all the time in the world, you can train yourself through the following simple exercises.

1. *Quiet your internal dialogue.* This is a simple way to contact the stillness that is the source of awareness. Sit quietly with your eyes closed. Let your breathing settle; put your attention in the center of your chest. As you inhale, let your consciousness settle on the syllable *So,* and exhale to the syllable *hum.* Feel the air coolly entering your body, gently carrying the sound; feel the air coolly leaving your body. *So-hum, So-hum.* (This is an ancient Indian mantra, but you can substitute *I am,* or *Amen,* or *Om,* and the result will be the same.)

   Continue for ten to twenty minutes. This simple meditation releases the mind from its incessant chattering. Three things may distract you: outside noises, sensations in your body, and distracting thoughts. When you notice any of these, just easily return to breathing on the sound *So-hum.* Don't try to maintain a rhythm; don't try to hypnotize yourself; this is an exercise in allowing the mind to find its own natural silence and effortless focus.

2. *Discharge tension.* Awareness, like water, is meant to flow easily, without interruption. When awareness becomes stuck, tension is created in the body. Cramps, pain, tightness, and stiffness are the most obvious symptoms of this, but at a deeper level your body is storing the memory of old stress. Yoga or deep energy work are great ways to release these body memories. Yet everyone's body has a natural mechanism for discharging tension, and you can take advantage of it immediately.

    Lie down before you go to sleep at night. Assume a position flat on your back without a pillow; spread your arms and legs at your side. Draw in a deep, slow breath, then release it through your mouth in a sigh, as freely and naturally as your body wants. Some sighs may be quick, almost like a gasp; others may be as deep as a sob. You may feel a sense of relief, sadness, grief, elation, or any other emotion. Be aware of the emotions as they arise; you are not just releasing physical tension; you are accessing bodily memories at the same time. The natural discharge of tension bundles thoughts, feelings, and sensations together, so let them all go at once. Do this exercise for no more than ten minutes, because it can be intense; allow yourself to fall asleep if your body wants to. That is also part of the discharge process.

3. *The purifying light.* When you are in the flow, there is a certain feeling associated with it: light, open, fresh. Being in this feeling gently pushes out negativity and resistance. One way to help this purifying process along is to bring light to the dark places that hide from being seen, where awareness has a hard time reaching. Visualizing inner light is the closest you can come to actually seeing awareness in its pure state; the real thing is invisible, yet when we say that someone is glowing with life, we are referring to the close relationship between life energy and awareness.

Sit or lie down, preferably not when you are so tired that you are ready to fall asleep. Turn your gaze inward, which means feel your body from the inside. Visualize a stream of gold-white light cascading down your body. The stream fills you from the crown of your head slowly through your chest, out your arms, then down your abdomen until it divides and flows down both legs. See the gold-white light go out through your feet and enter the ground.

Now take the light back up your body, this time using blue light. See the blue light start at your feet and slowly fill your body until it exits through the top of your head—see it form a laser beam going as high as you can see, out into space and beyond.

This whole cycle should take about one minute. Repeat ten times.

A simple variation is to sit quietly and breathe in the light, then slowly breathe it out. You can alternate between blue and gold-white, but finish by filling your entire body with gold light, seeing it suffuse everywhere, extending beyond you as a golden aura. Ask to be enclosed in this light for the rest of the day.

4. *Toning.* Sound can also be a powerful tool for moving stuck energy. Physical sensations and emotions are linked to sound. Sadness gives rise to weeping, happiness to laughter. These are the "sound signatures" of an underlying energy, and if you can find the signature, you can connect to the energy. Old, stuck energies are easier to find this way than trying to trace back the time and place where something happened in the past. Here's an exercise that uses sound to locate and release hidden energy:

Sit or lie down, preferably in a private place where you can feel comfortable making noise. Take a slow, easy, deep breath and see it reaching down below your diaphragm into the abdomen as deep as it can go. (Don't force it; just follow the breathing sensation.)

As you exhale, make a low tone. You want it to be long and steady–begin by humming a low note if that helps, but you want to do this with your mouth open. Let the tone extend for as long as you can, until your breath runs out. See this tone rising from your abdomen and coming out of your mouth. *Om* is an effective tone, but you aren't trying to sing or chant. Rather, you want your deep stresses to emerge on the tone. The secret here is to let your body make the tone it wants to make.

Toning takes practice. You have to do two things at once: make a tone and keep your awareness in your body. Don't pay undue attention to the tone itself. Let it come naturally. A good example is deep sighing. When you sigh and make a vocal noise at the same time, a groan or moan, for example, the two are combined. You feel how much physical relief the sigh is bringing as you make a natural, unconscious sound.

With practice you can locate many sound signatures connected to repressed feelings and buried experiences. Your body knows whether it wants to release a moan, groan, wail, scream, squeal, or cry. Instead of erupting all at once, which can feel jarring, you can provide a long tone that provides a more cushioned release. For example, a low, moaning sound accesses the whole lower abdominal region. A high-pitched *eeee* accesses the head. If you experiment, you will soon find which tone fits which energy. There is no limit to toning, once you have learned the knack of letting your body discharge tension by letting the stuck energy ride out smoothly and continuously on a sound.

RESURRECTING YOUR SOUL

THE SOUL IS YOUR
SPIRITUAL BODY

Having a soul could be the most useful thing in your life. So far, however, usefulness hasn't been the soul's major attribute. We are told that the soul is our link to God, but like God, it is invisible and far removed from daily affairs. Does your soul keep you healthy? Does it help you make decisions or resolve a crisis? All our lives we have referred to the soul with reverence, a tone of voice we wouldn't use to talk about our cars. In reality, however, most people get much farther in their cars than they ever do with their souls.

The soul has no function because it hasn't been successfully defined. No one is waiting for the world's religions to agree among themselves. It might seem as if the Buddhists are right to take a completely practical view—they dispense with the soul altogether, arguing that if it can't be defined, the soul has no reality. But that position isn't satisfying to the millions of people who believe that they have souls. (After all, we know we have a mind even though no two philosophers agree on a definition of that, either.) We can resurrect the soul from its dormant state by turning the tables: Instead of defining the soul first and asking what it does later, why not look at the need the soul fulfills first and worry about a strict definition later?

The main thing your soul does has already been mentioned: it connects you to God. In a sense the soul is like a step-down transformer. The electricity being sent through high-tension power lines is hundreds of times too powerful to go directly into your house; it would burn out every circuit in a flash. In the same way, the ultimate spiritual power can't surge directly into you and me without harm. It must be stepped down and adapted to human life. The soul exists to perform that function.

I realize that this description seemingly depends upon the existence of God, but it doesn't need to. Without resorting to any religious belief, we know that the universe contains almost infinite amounts of energy, and yet Nature has found a way to step down the heat of the nearest star, which burns at millions of degrees Celsius, to support life on our planet. It has stepped down the force of gravity, which is so condensed at the heart of a black hole that time and space are sucked out of existence, so that it has only enough force to hold the human body together. Finally, the electromagnetism that explodes in a bolt of lightning—explosions that once struck the earth's surface millions of times a day in the planet's infancy—has been stepped down to the minuscule electrical firings of brain cells, which are so weak that it takes extremely precise instruments even to detect them. (The brain's entire electrical potential is about the equivalent of a sixty-watt lightbulb, but this charge is subdivided among 100 billion neurons, making each brain cell's portion infinitesimal, a matter of microvolts.)

If the physical forces of the universe must be stepped down so dramatically to work on a human scale, it seems possible that God can be thought of as a universal force that must also be stepped down. But *force* is a materialistic term. When we think of God, we use terms like *love, compassion, truth, intelligence,* and *creativity.* However much they disagree, every spiritual tradition sees these qualities on a scale from zero to infinite. Inert objects do not exhibit love or compassion; they have no visible intelligence. That's the zero end of the scale. Human beings are imbued with love, compassion, and intelligence, and as we look around, we believe that these qualities are visible in other living creatures. That's the middle region of the scale.

Then we project a higher reality where love and compassion become unconditional, where intelligence is so vast that it can run the universe, and where creativity can bring the universe into being. That's the highest end of the scale, and the most contentious.

Science doesn't acknowledge higher reality, because once you look beyond the human brain an invisible region begins. You can see a neuron and therefore claim that intelligence begins with it, but since a neuron is only made of atoms, how exactly did an atom acquire intelligence? Not to mention the aspects of the mind we most cherish—love, compassion, truth, and all the other qualities that give life meaning.

The soul serves to get us past the blocks put up by materialism, but, surprisingly, at the same time it also gets us past the faith demanded by religion. The obstacle put up by science is that everything must be material; the obstacle put up by religion is that one must believe in invisible forces without always having direct proof that they exist. As we will see, the soul can be mapped, even though it is invisible. The human body is a complex system of energy and awareness, and the soul can be defined as a subtler version of those two ingredients. Functioning as your spiritual body, the soul generates and organizes the energy of love, the energy of compassion, the awareness of truth, the awareness of creativity and intelligence. In that way it fulfills needs that are just as basic as the need of the physical body for food and oxygen.

A complete map of the soul would be at least as complex as the human brain. However, here's a simple map that will turn out to be extremely useful.

GOD = *infinite* energy, love, creativity, intelligence

SOUL = *stepping down* energy, love, creativity, intelligence

MIND/BODY = *human level* of energy, love, creativity, intelligence

A glance at this diagram suggests an exciting possibility: the soul can bring even more of God into the human realm. For millions of people, God's infinite love has been stepped down too far. They experience only a fraction of the love they should, and even that love comes and goes; it sometimes weakens to the point that their lives seem to have no love at all. The same is true of intelligence and creativity. Millions of people function day to day using the same routines, the same conditioning from the past, the same fixed reactions. Yet there is no reason to believe that God's infinite qualities must be so diminished when they reach the human level. Looking around, we see countless examples of people who possess enormous reserves of love, creativity, and intelligence. The existence of a Saint Francis, an Einstein, or a Leonardo da Vinci indicates that human potential can reach amazing heights. Why and how did their souls step down so that so much potential still came through—a gush of genius—while for other people the step-down yields barely a trickle?

The answer lies at the level of the soul. Just as physical disease can be traced back to distorted energy patterns at a subtle level of the body, any limitation of the mind can be traced back to distortions of energy, only the level is even subtler, the level of the soul. Not that we want to isolate the mind. The body's energy is dependent on the mind, and once we find out why our thoughts, beliefs, wishes, and aspirations are not being fulfilled, removing those obstacles will serve to liberate the body even more.

Speaking personally, I find a great emotional release when the soul becomes a practical aspect of life. "Who am I, and why am I here?" The two questions go hand in hand. To answer them, religion says, "You're a child of God, and you are here to reflect God's glory." Science says, "You're a complex lump of molecules, and you are here to do what those molecules dictate." Both answers have produced as much trouble and misery as they have alleviated.

Religion is disturbing because it seems optimistic on the surface but deeply pessimistic underneath. What could be more optimistic than seeing yourself as a child of God? You fit into a divine plan stretching back to the dawn of creation. As this plan unfolds (in the Christian West, at least), it will redeem every soul that loves God. Underlying this scheme is dark pessimism, however, because God may hate us for our sins, and even when we strain not to disobey divine commandments, we unwittingly make mistakes. Worse, the divine plan seems to allow room for immense pain and suffering that God either can't or won't prevent. Our purpose in life comes down to guesswork and desperate hopes that we don't fall into disgrace. Who can find the light when the path lies in the dark? Perhaps the plan is knowable only to God.

The other ready-made answer, proposed by science, is disturbing for the opposite reason. It is pessimistic on the surface and has just enough optimism underneath to keep us from losing hope. Science denies that life has any purpose. Existence is trapped between inflexible laws (gravity, entropy, the weak forces) on one hand and randomness on the other. The most cherished aspects of life, such as love and beauty, are reduced to random chemical firings in the brain. The most valued behavior, such as self-sacrifice and altruism, comes down to genetic mutations that have no purpose other than survival. Taken at face value, no one would choose to live according to such a fixed, meaningless worldview, but science provides a mitigating layer of optimism with its belief in progress. If we are learning more day by day, so if technology makes life easier with each new invention, the pessimism of science can be ignored. You can turn up your iPod if the void begins to seem intolerable.

A clear path to your soul is available, but just as we've seen with the body, drastically new thinking is required. We need a new set of breakthroughs, each one rooted in a new reality that isn't bound by the flawed materialism of science or the flawed idealism of religion. Are you meant to be more loving and creative, happier and wiser? Some people do become more loving as their lives unfold, but others turn in the opposite direction. Some people become wiser, while others cling to ignorant beliefs. Opposites keep clashing. We take the bitter with the sweet because we have to. What this indicates is that there are just as many breakdowns in the nonphysical part of life as the physical. Each breakthrough will take us past these breakdowns. At the same time we will acquire true knowledge of the soul to replace mere wishful thinking. Reaching the soul means fulfilling the deepest aspirations of the human heart.

Bringing spirit down to earth

Religion made a terrible mistake when it consigned the body to the "lower" physical world while the soul was lifted to the "higher" spiritual realm. A functioning soul is not so very different from a functioning body. Both are involved in the same things—awareness and energy—that make life possible. "I am my body" and "I am my soul" are two faces of the same truth. The problem is that we have lost contact with the soul. It wasn't created to be useless; we made it that way.

Imagine yourself sitting in a doctor's office, waiting nervously for your appointment. Your eye is distracted by a rose garden outside the window, or a solitary tree. Consider how these plants live. A seed begins to grow, and inside the seed is the plant's entire life. As it grows, a rose or a tree isn't tempted to deviate from its programmed existence. In harmony with its environment, a rose effortlessly expresses its beauty, and a tree its strength. Human beings, however, are not tied to a preset plan. We have more latitude to shape our own destiny.

Somewhere along the way, we used that free will to make a choice to divide the body from the soul. The body became identified with sin, and the soul with God; the body with Earth, and the soul with Heaven. But if you take a functional approach, there's no need for such a division. We don't say that roses have a body and a soul. Everything about them, from the subtlest information in their genes to the prick of their thorns, unfolds as one life. A rose's perfection— so rich, velvet, aromatic, and intensely colored—is present here and now. The same is true of you, if you can get past the split that cuts your soul off from daily life.

There is no reason for anyone to dream of a lost Paradise, a garden from which the first man and woman were banished. Paradise moved inside us to become a vision of infinite possibilities. Your chance to evolve is right here, right this minute, in this very body. Your soul can step down much more of God's perfection than you can even imagine. The limited degree of love, intelligence, and creativity that you experience in your life barely hints at the untapped possibilities.

To resurrect your soul, you must do the opposite of what your past conditioning tells you to. Instead of turning to a higher power, you turn to yourself. Instead of leaving your body behind, you take it on the spiritual journey. Instead of condemning physical desire and temptation, you follow desire into the unknown region where the soul resides.

It's strange to say, but even when you lost contact with your soul, your body didn't. Cells keep the faith. They have been using "higher" awareness since you were born. Here's a practical example: It's become a medical cliché that we use only 10 percent of our brains. In a sense this claim is a trick, because the 90 percent that isn't being used wasn't made for thinking. There are billions of cells known as *glia* (Greek for "glue") that surround your brain cells to hold them in place. Glia outnumber neurons about ten to one. For a long time they were viewed as second-class citizens in the brain, serving as little more than structural reinforcement, like rebar in cement. No one suspected the glia's secret role, which turned out to make for a fascinating spectacle. Glia are like starbursts or hedgehogs, with dozens of tiny strands emanating from their centers.

When an embryo in the womb is ready to develop a brain, there's a huge challenge ahead. How can a few hundred or thousand stem cells turn into the billions of brain cells required? It's not sufficient for stem cells to divide madly until they reach the right number (although they do that, too). The brain has many parts, and the neurons responsible for sight or hearing, for example, must get to their proper locations, while other neurons responsible for emotions and higher thinking must get to their proper destination, too.

To do that, each stem cell goes on a migration. The journey is often as long, relatively speaking, as the flight of the arctic tern, which flies almost from pole to pole. In the stem cell's case, it can migrate almost from one end of the embryo to the other. Migrating stem cells line up by the millions, nose to tail, and travel along the strands of the glia. Under a powerful microscope you can view their journey and marvel at how the stem cells that need to go to one region turn off the main highway and follow the exact glial strand that leads to their final home, while the next bunch of stem cells takes a different turn. Each move is purposeful and guided. The brain grows from the inside out, so newcomers travel past older brain cells to form layer after layer of tissue. When researchers discovered that glia served as guides for this incredibly complex process, their reputation grew enormously. It grew even more when it was found that after serving as guides, glia can turn into brain cells themselves.

In what way is this not a spiritual journey? Stem cells are being guided home by a higher intelligence, acquiring wisdom along the way. Your life has been following the same hidden pattern, but instead of following glistening glial strands, you are guided by your soul. It holds the blueprint of God's intentions just as a blueprint on paper holds an architect's intentions. Everything a cell can do must come from somewhere. It would be foolish to believe that brain cells act randomly; otherwise, stem cells would float about aimlessly with nowhere to go. Our best proof that brain cells are aware and intelligent is that they *act* aware and intelligent.

But the soul isn't confined to stem-cell journeys happening under the dark cover of the skull. Your soul brings guidance from the outside as well as the inside. You can sit in a chair and reach a life-changing insight, or a great teacher can walk in the room to deliver it. One event takes place inside you, the other outside. But both are events that alter awareness. Once you reconnect with your soul, you aren't restricted to only a few levels of existence: they all open up to the same ever-expanding consciousness. And at every level there is guidance.

The brain connection

The most practical way to think of the soul is as a connector. But if that is what your soul is doing, connecting you to subtle, invisible levels of life, there have to be junction points with your body. In particular, we need brain connections. As it stands, the brain is the great obstacle to the soul. Neurologists don't feel the need for any invisible explanations for love. They can exhibit brain scans showing that various areas of the cortex and limbic system light up in lovers that don't light up in the rest of us; being in love comes down to bursts of electricity and chemicals, just as, for the geneticist, being in love comes down to a love gene (as yet undiscovered, but the search goes on).

It's up to us, then, to prove that love comes from a higher place. If we don't want to accept that the brain creates love out of an electrochemical soup inside the skull, where's the evidence that it comes from anywhere else? Let's turn back to the example of the Tibetan Buddhist monks who developed "compassionate brains" as the result of practicing a meditation on compassion. A spiritual quality was transformed into physical manifestation. The split between body and soul was erased. In Sanskrit the same word, *Daya*, applies to both compassion and the everyday trait of sympathy. It turns out that the brain is extremely variable when it comes to sympathy. Functional MRIs taken inside a New Mexico prison (the only program of its type) show that inmates who score high on tests for psychopathic tendencies also have distorted brain function. Psychopaths possess the least innate sympathy imaginable. They have no conscience; they can commit acts of terrible cruelty without feeling a shred of the pain they are inflicting. Watching the blood ooze from a knife wound is an indifferent act, like watching juice ooze from a steak.

Can a psychopath's brain be turned into a compassionate brain? No one knows; the psychiatric profession has largely given up changing psychopaths either through drugs or conventional couch therapy. But we do know that the brain is malleable enough that it embraces every moral state, and that every state of consciousness requires a shift in the brain. Just thinking that you are compassionate doesn't do the job, which leads me to conclude that compassion isn't a mood, a moral teaching, an ethical obligation, or a social ideal. It's a subtle activity of the brain that needs that subtle level to exist. On its own, the brain can't produce change; it merely adapts to your intention. This gives us a slightly more sophisticated map of what the soul is doing as it steps down subtle energy to the human scale. Take anything that you want out of life. Your soul contains the potential for it to come true. Your mind brings the potential to the level of wishing, dreaming, wanting, and desiring. Your brain then produces the result; you learn how to achieve what you want.

Here's the whole scheme reduced to a simple formulation:

Soul carries the *potential*
Mind carries the *intention*
Brain produces the *result*

This is the basic flow chart of life. It reverses the flow that science espouses, where everything must begin in the brain. But there's no reason why the physical level has to be primary. The brain learns new skills by forming neural networks, but the desire for change itself must come from somewhere else. If you think of compassion as a skill, like learning to play the violin, it must be prompted by wanting to learn compassion in the first place. This gives us an insight into the soul's most useful role: it motivates us to reach higher.

A useful soul gives you the vision, the desire, and the will to evolve. Your mind carries that vision into the realm of thinking and wanting. Your brain receives the message and begins to give it physical shape. This process is already familiar to anyone who has learned a new skill.

But when we learn to do anything now, we are only conscious of thinking and wanting. The brain isn't accessible, since we don't dip into it and start rewiring its connections by hand. The physical level takes care of itself once we start thinking. The soul level is also inaccessible. We don't ask God how to ride a bicycle. Only in the isolated compartment we call spirit, where prayers occur, do we say that we are asking God. There is no need for such isolation. Every skill, from the most mundane to one as exalted as compassion, follows the same process. It's a mental process that reverberates through the body and soul at the same time.

Here are the steps involved:

1. Becoming genuinely interested.
2. Pursuing your interest spontaneously.
3. Practicing until you see improvement.
4. Sticking with your practice until the new skill is mastered.

Simple as these steps are, they require input from awareness; the whole process can't be triggered simply by the brain. Step 1, becoming genuinely interested, requires inspiration. To be interested in compassion isn't an ordinary occurrence in a society driven by self-gratification, even among mature, psychologically developed people. But if you read the lore of compassion that infuses Buddhism and Christianity, inspiration arises naturally. The same can happen when you are moved by compassionate acts performed in brave rescues, or by relief missions to places where people are suffering.

Step 2, pursuing your interest spontaneously, requires turning inward, because the inner landscape is the country of compassion. Once you find the place of empathy inside you, it wants to express itself. Empathy may bring discomfort (the very word *compassion* means "to suffer with"), so you have to overcome your natural urge to turn away from someone else's distress. Yet in some people compassion triggers a unique kind of joy that they want to follow.

Step 3, practicing until you see improvement, requires discipline, because you must constantly renew your dedication in the face of old conditioning that tempts you to turn away from compassion in pursuit of the ego's constant demands. Pleasure is innately selfish; therefore, no one finds compassion without a struggle.

Step 4, sticking with your practice until the new skill is mastered, requires patience, because there are many inner forces—and outer ones, too—that oppose compassion. Higher awareness doesn't force change; it melts away old patterns so that new ones can replace them, which takes time. (Ask aid workers who have flown to a disaster in the developing world. Their idealism vanishes at the first shocking sight of real devastation. They pass through stages of despair, frustration, and numbness. Yet beneath the surface a new strength develops, one that not only adjusts to the outer spectacle of suffering, but blossoms into a much stronger empathy.)

This outline gives us more insight into what I've called "subtle action," which begins in awareness and then reaches into the body. Subtle action erases the boundary between a compassionate person and a compassionate brain. Each needs the other; neither is enough on its own. Heretical as it may sound, it took subtle action to create Buddha and Christ. They established unshakable compassion in themselves by following the same steps an ordinary person would follow. Buddha and Christ didn't realize, perhaps, that they had to transform their brains, but they were certain that higher awareness was at work. At the very least, to be compassionate while *not* changing the brain is a temporary achievement, subject to the winds of change. Because we were all born with the capacity to sympathize, our brains await their next instruction to expand this capacity to the level of the soul.

Garry's story

The subtle level of the mind, which connects with the soul, is attuned to signs, omens, portents, suggestions, pointers, and prophecy—indicators of the built-in guidance that is inherent in life. Conscious thinking doesn't have to be involved. But we are so used to thinking as the brain's highest function that it's easy to overlook the silent, hidden aspects of the mind until they suddenly make themselves known. Then it's no longer possible to overlook them any longer.

"I became a seeker when my career suddenly collapsed," recalls Garry, who is forty-five and was diagnosed with a serious heart valve defect in his early thirties. "I went through a difficult surgery that led to complications. Recovery took a long time. The other guys who had been my friends on the fast track after business school dropped me; it was like my problems had made me somehow different. And they were right. I wasn't like them anymore. Things were shifting inside.

"I took to wandering around town, waiting for something but not knowing what. One day I was getting on a bus, and I had the thought, *Am I doing the right thing with my life?* The man in front of me, a complete stranger, turned around and said, 'Trust it.' Then, as if he hadn't said anything, he got on the bus without another word. That moment began a series of strange incidents. I was walking past a kid carrying a boom box, and at that moment I was thinking of going back to my old job. Suddenly he turned up the volume, and the song that blasted at me was 'No, no, no, Delilah.'

"I laughed, but I wasn't entirely amused. I felt a spooky connection with something beyond me. Soon afterwards I decided to go to a tarot card reader, and when I asked the cards if I should go on a spiritual path, the best card in the deck came up—it showed ten golden cups with a rainbow overhead and a joyous crowd dancing down below. After a while it got so I could ask myself a question and turn on the TV, knowing that the next words coming out of the set would answer my question."

"And it never failed?" I asked.

Garry smiled. "Only when I tried to control it. The whole phenomenon had a certain innocence and surprise factor, so most of the time I was caught off guard. If I tried to push things or manipulate the outcome, nothing happened."

"Did you get deep answers?" I asked.

He shook his head. "Not always, but each one fit the moment. It was very personal, speaking directly to my situation."

Garry had more examples to relate, as everyone does who finds that his life is guided. No one is especially chosen for guidance. It is an aspect of life that permeates every level, for all of us. Certainly the instincts built into so-called lower creatures are a profound form of guidance. One observes salmon, for example, who live for years in the open ocean and then return to spawn in the exact same stream where they were born. Their unerring guidance is explained by smell—it is presumed that even hundreds of miles out at sea they can detect molecules of water from their native freshwater birthplace. But something more holistic is also at work, because salmon don't respond to this smell until they reach a certain age, at which time they find the right direction, change color, stop eating, and begin to secrete large amounts of cortisol, a hormone that will increase to the point that it kills every fish soon after spawning. Timing, chemistry, sex drive, and life expectancy are precisely coordinated by an inner guidance that remains mysterious.

In Sanskrit the inner guidance that shapes a human life is called *Upaguru,* "the teacher who is near." Over the past four decades the word *guru* has become familiar in the West to describe a spiritual teacher—the root word means "dispeller of darkness." In other words, anyone who can guide you to see what you need to see serves as your guru. No one's spiritual journey is shaped by a cookie cutter. Each is made up of individual moments that occur only once in the entire history of the universe. It takes infinite flexibility for your soul to understand what you need at any given moment. But every soul is up to the challenge, and therefore each daily moment contains, hidden inside it, a small, unique revelation. Zen Buddhists hold that every question already contains its own answer. Your soul takes the same perspective.

Awareness has the magical ability to merge question and answer. In Garry's case, as soon as he posed a dilemma, a chance event or a casually overheard phrase would contain the solution. Without being aware, he would never have put the two together—you have to notice a connection before a coincidence turns into synchronicity. Someone who is unaware won't notice that he is being guided. You may be surprised when a perfect stranger tells you exactly what you need to know and skeptical that it means anything. Yet who hasn't opened a book at random, only to find that the information he wanted was on that page? (I know a legally blind scholar who told me with a note of triumph that on a good day he didn't need to use the library's microfiche catalog. He would go into the stacks and be guided to the exact book he needed, even to the point that he could pull a volume down at random only to discover that it was the right one.)

Upaguru is a mystical phenomenon only if you assume that awareness is limited to the brain; asking a question "in here" can't produce an answer "out there." But the wall between inner and outer reality is artificial. Awareness is everywhere in nature. Seeing how animals are guided, it's hard to maintain skepticism on that point. Migrating whales pick up calls from their kind hundreds of miles away; migrating monarch butterflies return to the same mountainous area in Mexico without fail, even though it is their first migration home after hatching. A breakthrough can occur when you accept that awareness is what guides you. If you attune yourself to that possibility, you are reconnecting to your soul, which is nothing but awareness in its most expanded form.

Relying on the soul

Awareness comes from the soul, yet many people would say that they have never been guided, much less transformed. For centuries human beings have prayed for signs that there is a higher power. These signs are actually everywhere, but there's a subtle difference between inner and outer guidance. One person's insight is another person's message from God. One person's glimpse of inner light is another person's angel. The realm of the soul has room for both.

External guidance comes to people for whom the best proof of spirit is physical. There's an enormous body of lore about a rescue squad of angels and protectors who come to earth in times of peril. Many of these are contemporary eyewitness accounts. Travelers who find themselves stranded on a deserted road in the midst of a howling storm suddenly see headlights. A kind stranger gets out and changes a tire, fixes a carburetor, or connects jumper cables. This helper then disappears around the next bend, and the grateful recipient reports an encounter with an angel.

I was vividly struck by a vignette on television in which a woman told her story of angelic intervention. She found herself alone one Christmas with no money and two young children to take care of. She despaired of telling her children that there would be no holiday for them that year, since she couldn't afford presents under the tree and a turkey dinner. On Christmas Day there was a knock on the door. A kindly neighbor invited the whole family to his apartment, where he provided a lavish spread and gifts for the children. The young mother, who had never seen this neighbor, was overwhelmed by his kindness. She knocked on his door a few days later to thank him, only to find that the apartment was empty. When she inquired at the manager's office to ask where the stranger had gone, she was informed that the apartment had gone unrented for months. The manager had never seen the stranger she was looking for.

In first-person accounts like this, belief and skepticism are both beside the point, I think. We have no hard-and-fast proof either way. Skeptics are forced to prove a negative, that angels don't exist. Believers are forced to produce an angel for the camera, and that, so far, hasn't been done convincingly. Even so, nothing is going to stem the constant flow of such stories. The deeper issue is that the spiritual world is kept at arm's length when it depends on angels. What happens when the angels don't show up? That's where inner guidance proves so valuable, because the world within is never far away.

Without the inner support that comes from your own awareness, you are left in a very vulnerable position. In one psychiatric case study, a middle-aged woman came for therapy in a very agitated state, unable to sleep and prey to fearful thoughts. A few months before, she had been happy and untroubled. But as she was walking out of a restaurant by herself one evening, a purse-snatcher ran up and grabbed her pocketbook. He barely laid hands on her, so she wasn't hurt physically. She had little of importance in her purse and lost only the small amount of money in her wallet.

The woman told herself that she was lucky to escape a violent mugging, but over the next few weeks, these rational reassurances crumbled. She began to feel unsafe for the first time in her life. She kept reliving the incident, and the images made her increasingly afraid. Most victims of muggings experience residual anxiety, no longer feeling quite as safe as they did before. But this woman fell into deeper anxiety. In therapy she discovered that she had been masking a profound fear of death. She had made herself feel safe by believing that she led a charmed life. For this woman, who was growing older and had never examined her youthful sense of immortality, one shock was enough to crack the fantasy of that charmed life. Then the way was opened for darker energies to pour out from their hiding place.

The irony of this story for me is that people *are* immortal. The fantasy of immortality masks the very thing that's true. The soul steps God down to the human level, which gives us the appearance of being mortal. But the soul *is* you. The fact that the soul exists gives us an aspect of the self that transcends the cycle of birth and death. We don't have to separate the lore of angels from the lore of the soul. We do have to break the supernatural spell that religion weaves around obedience, faith, and theological dogma. Under that spell, people lose the ability to find their own inner guidance, which never sleeps and is always at hand.

To break this spell, you must rely on personal experience. The soul can be tested. You can ask your soul to produce results by running your own soul-experiment. In fact, all of the breakthroughs in this part of the book are self-experiments to prove that higher awareness can be trusted. If your first experiment has positive results, you can try another, and then another. This is the most practical way to resurrect the soul. The more useful the soul becomes, the more real it is, not as religious dogma but as a part of yourself.

In Your Life: Guided by the Soul

If your inner guide is always with you, why aren't you aware of it? Actually, you are. Every desire pushes you in a certain direction. Every thought looks forward or backward. Anyone who has a purpose in life, even if that purpose is limited to getting through the day, is following his or her own inner guidance. The real issue is how wise this guidance is. Your soul has the potential to be a perfect guide. You must first attune your mind to a subtler level, and then your brain will adapt—this is the flow of life that governs all change. Being guided is a process, and at this moment you find yourself somewhere—the beginning, middle, or end—of that process.

In the beginning, you catch just a few glimpses of subtle guidance. Usually these seem like chance events or lucky coincidences. You find that you have made a decision that benefited you, but unlike your usual everyday choices, this decision has a certain sense of rightness about it, as if it were meant to be. We've all had that feeling at one time or another. You then have a choice, either to say, "I had the strangest feeling that this was meant to happen," after which you put the whole thing out of your mind, or to stop and look more closely at what happened. How you make the choice determines whether you will begin to listen to your guidance or not.

In the middle of the process, your questioning has become more urgent and important. You have seen repeatedly that various situations came out in your favor. Instead of settling for a vague feeling that God was on your side, or that fate smiled at you for a moment, you became more actively involved. You ask more personal questions: Why did this happen to me? Who or what is watching over me? Am I the one who's doing this? There's no guarantee that you will come up with the same answers as the *rishis*, the sages of India. They concluded that the higher self, which we are calling the soul, is the source of everything, including God and fate.

Today, most people fence-sit. While some develop a confirmed conviction that God is rewarding them and therefore must be worshipped, others consider God a vague belief that doesn't impinge on everyday life; divine reward, after all, raises the specter of divine punishment. In a secular world, cause and effect don't operate on such a supernatural basis. By fence-sitting, a person can worry about God sending bad things their way, while at the same time using practical means to gain success and avoid failure.

The end of the process comes when you stop fence-sitting. You no longer halfheartedly believe in God and fate, but you seize the reins yourself. At this point, guidance becomes an acknowledged part of you and the journey you are consciously taking. You see the truth of *Upaguru*—there is guidance at every moment, because the guru is inside yourself. The teacher is as near as your next breath. When I call this the end of the process, I don't mean that it reaches a halt, but rather that it matures. The process of being guided is fully revealed, at which point you take full advantage of it.

How do you get to this point?

1. Realize that you are on a journey to higher consciousness, and embrace it.
2. Expand your awareness, through meditation, contemplation, and other means.
3. Ask for guidance, simply and sincerely, and then wait for it to appear.
4. Trust your finest instincts. Guidance doesn't come in the form of fear, premonition, omens, distrust, or self-importance. All of those things exist around us; they cloud our view of true guidance, which is always a signpost to the next step of personal growth.

The last point is extremely important but also tricky. All of us have reacted afterwards to a bad event by saying, "I just knew that was going to happen. I had this bad feeling." But that isn't guidance. It's the voice of anxiety having an I-told-you-so moment. The difference is that true guidance is never fearful. Your soul doesn't say, "Watch out, bad things are about to happen." It steers you out of the situation *before* things turn bad. Sometimes it guides you out of danger before there's even the slightest hint of it. The voice of fear never does that, since it reacts to immediate threat, real or imagined. Getting past the voice of fear is important, because fear is part of the shield that keeps you from your inner self. Like the fantasy of being protected, fear is the fantasy that you are always in danger. True guidance removes these fantasies and replaces them with reality: you possess a guide inside; it can be trusted. To activate this reality, we will go deeper into how the soul connects to the everyday self.

The connecting link is the mind, and much depends on whether your mind is open to your soul or closed to it. In a state of complete openness, the mind can realize infinite possibilities, far beyond guidance and protection. In its closed state, however, the mind mistakes reality. It creates a world that's random, impersonal, and unsafe. Because each of us unthinkingly starts off in that world, our most urgent business is to crack the shell of illusion. Higher consciousness stands ready to deliver the gifts promised in every spiritual tradition as grace and Providence. In the flow of life, those gifts are meant to be yours, effortlessly and constantly.

Breakthrough #1

There's an Easier Way to Live

The first soul breakthrough takes something that used to be difficult and makes it easy. Connecting with your soul is as easy as breathing, and just as natural. When pollsters ask, "Do you believe you have a soul?" close to 90 percent of respondents say yes. But that statistic is misleading, because very few people have actually experienced their souls. They avoid the spiritual journey because they assume it will be arduous, with many sacrifices along the way. But doesn't that describe everyday life already? (One of the major bestsellers of the eighties, M. Scott Peck's *The Road Less Traveled*, hooked millions of readers with three simple words: "Life is difficult.")

Connecting to your soul is actually easier than whatever you are doing right now. It takes effort to keep your soul at a distance. When you stop struggling, the path to the soul is automatic. Everything you want to achieve will naturally unfold. This is what Jesus meant when he said, "Ask, and you shall receive. Knock, and the door will be opened."

When you meet with day-to-day obstacles, you have put up inner obstacles first. These obstacles block the flow of life from soul to mind to body. If the flow hadn't been blocked, it would bring everything the soul has to offer. The soul provides an open channel. If you ask for the truth about something, the truth dawns. If you ask for the solution to a problem, the solution appears. That's why Buddhism teaches that every question is paired with its answer at the very moment the question arises.

If any channel in awareness is closed off, it has been temporarily blocked. The trap is that so much of this blockage happens without being noticed. We have all adapted to "life is difficult" because we saw no alternative. Like plaque building up on artery walls until the whole blood vessel is clogged, the buildup of struggle and strain happens by tiny degrees.

I was reminded of this when I was waiting in an airport between flights. It was several years ago. My daughter Mallika had a two-year-old girl, Tara, my first grandchild. I often eased the boredom of airports by calling Tara on my cell phone. It became a ritual that delighted both of us, me because Tara recognized my voice, and her because to a two-year-old a telephone is a magical toy.

This time when I hung up I noticed a frazzled young woman rushing toward me to catch her flight. She had two toddlers in tow, and what with being late and struggling with luggage and a stroller, the mother was overwhelmed. This in turn caused her children to cry. I saw her drag them to the check-in counter. But the young woman was out of luck. The gate had closed, and she would have to wait for the next flight. She pleaded that she had to get home to her family. You could tell that she was at her wits' end after a long day.

But the agent at the counter was firm. Rules were rules. Passengers had to arrive at the gate at least fifteen minutes before their flight. Frustrated, her kids still crying, the young mother dragged herself away. When she was out of earshot, the agent turned to her assistant and said, "What could I do? My hands are tied." The assistant agent was still watching the young mother. "I guess things are tough all over," she said, shaking her head.

Life is a baffling mixture of Tara's innocent joy—and the joy she inspired in me—and constant struggle like that of the young mother. We don't see ourselves choosing one over the other, and yet we do. For each of us was like Tara when life began. The tragedy is that we learn to struggle so young, too young to realize that innocence and simplicity should never have been abandoned. Only in innocence can you receive the gifts of the soul. Once you accept that you are supposed to struggle in order to survive, that presumption becomes your reality. It gathers its own energy and momentum. Your brain quickly learns to conform. Once your brain is conditioned, the look, feel, and sound of the world have been fixed—until you escape that conditioning.

Tuning in to your soul

We already know that the body is aware. By tuning in to it, you can increase its awareness. Tuning in is also how you clear a channel to the soul. You are tuning in to your soul anytime you choose to grow and expand. On the other hand, when you tune out, the soul connection is blocked. Anytime you choose to contract in your awareness, the channel to your soul is squeezed shut. Everyone experiences both states. As mystically as we talk about the soul, being connected to it comes down to everyday experience.

Tuned In

Things are going easily for me.
I'm calmly certain.
The answer is clear.
Everything fits together.
I feel in harmony with the situation.
There are no outer obstacles.
Opposites are reconciled.
I'm open to any possibility.
I don't judge myself or others.
I am whole.

Whenever you are jarred out of this state, you are no longer connected to your soul. This condition also comes down to everyday experience.

Tuned Out

Things aren't going smoothly for me.
I'm confused and uncertain.
The answer isn't clear. I go back and forth.

Everything is mixed up.

I feel out of sync with the situation.

There are many obstacles.

I'm conflicted inside.

I find it hard to see a way out.

I keep blaming myself, and others.

I feel incomplete. I must be lacking something.

Please don't take these two opposites as either absolute or permanent. Each of us tunes in and out every day. Our awareness contracts under stress, much like the body's stress response. Our aim here is to achieve a permanent connection that can't be broken, yet even short of that, people reach moments of very profound connection that change their lives.

A friend recently told me about an incident from his past that illustrates the point. It was a moment when his awareness expanded all at once.

"I was bumming around Europe with a backpack. I was twenty-six, and my life was a permanent vacation. I held temp jobs for just long enough to bankroll another trip.

"On this occasion I was the last person to get on the plane as a standby. I plunked myself down next to a man reading a book. Neither of us looked at the other. The plane took off, and I sat there. For some reason I had this empty feeling, accompanied by a vague dissatisfaction. I was surprised because, in general, bumming around Europe had been the happiest phase of my life. But at that moment I heard myself asking, *What are you doing? This is a total waste.*

"All at once I noticed that the man next to me had put down his book and was looking my way. 'Is something wrong?' he said. I was startled, but for some reason I didn't brush the question off. The guy seemed sympathetic, so I told him what was happening. He asked me if I wanted his opinion. I said sure. 'You've come to a moment of decision,' he said.

"I never expected that. 'What kind of decision?' I said.

" 'You're considering leaving your childhood behind.'

"He kind of smiled, but I knew he was serious. 'How do you know that?' I asked.

" 'Because it happened to me,' he said. 'One day it just dawned on me. *I'm an adult.* I had crossed a line, and there was no going back. I think the same thing just happened to you.' "

My friend shook his head. "He was right. I didn't even have to struggle with it that much. My adolescence was over. I flew home. I put my backpack away in the attic. I gave up my temp jobs and got serious on the work front."

"Those aren't unusual things," I pointed out.

"I know. Everyone has to grow up sometime. But wasn't it strange that it happened to me all at once, and that I was sitting next to someone who knew what I was going through, and had experienced the exact same moment?"

This is an example of how higher awareness reaches into everyday life. On the surface your mind is completely occupied with thinking and feeling. A rush of sensations and ideas fills your head from the moment you wake up. But life has hidden patterns that awaken in much the same way that a dormant gene will suddenly become activated. Out of the blue you have a realization, and in a moment your whole life can change.

Most of the time, however, changing the trajectory of your life is less dramatic. It's a process that unfolds according to its own rhythm and timing. But whether fast or slow, realizations are mysterious events. You discover that you know something you didn't know before. An old perspective suddenly gives way to a new one. Psychologists have given us broad maps of major life changes, such as the "identity crisis" that turns teenagers into adults sometime in their early to mid-twenties. There is also the "midlife crisis" when the end of young adulthood creates panic and generates a powerful impulse to be young a second time around.

The significant feature of any turning point is that the meaning of life changes. And when it does, the change can be stunningly drastic, like Scrooge turning from total selfishness to total altruism on Christmas Day. When you suddenly fall in and out of love, when you suddenly find religion after decades of unbelief, or when you go to work and discover that overnight a fulfilling career has become empty, a major change in awareness has occurred. If the meaning of life shifts profoundly, higher awareness has reached into your life from the level of the soul.

Take the experience of love. Love is most overwhelming as a physical and emotional state, which is how we experience it in the visible world. To be in love is to be aroused by the sexual and romantic thrill of another person: your beloved. The heart pounds, and the pulse races. The mundane activities of everyday life pale compared to the intoxication of falling in love. If you try to refine this tumult while it's washing over you, you can't. But in calmer moments, love is more stable and pure, as in the love between mother and child. If we keep refining it, a love for humanity—known as compassion—arises. Purer still is the love based on abstraction, such as love of beauty or love of truth. Finally, for those few who reach the subtlest essence, love becomes an aspect of God. Not all love reaches this exalted goal. The point is the process, the refining of awareness until it becomes more delicate, subtle, and pure. You will still love your beloved—the physical aspect of life doesn't disappear—but at the same time you will feel the higher aspects of love. It's as if you live in the body and see through it at the same time.

To tune in to your soul, you must participate in this process of purification. Many of us have lost our ability to do that, however, which makes it seem only natural that the soul feels abstract, remote, wispy, and aloof. People began to speak of it as "the ghost in the machine," a phrase that coupled two false notions, since the soul isn't a ghost and the body isn't a machine. This disconnect isn't about sin or disobedience. You didn't commit a terrible crime that caused you to be punished as a lost soul (I realize that committed Christians would fiercely argue this point, but in a secular society it seems evident that most people don't feel that they have inherited a mortal sin from Adam and Eve).

Even if you are a devout Christian, it's fascinating to note that in the Old Testament, God promises to send a messenger to earth, one who will bring the Lord into the temple, using these words: "*Who shall abide the day of his coming? For he will be like a refiner's fire or a launderer's soap. He will sit as a refiner and purifier of silver.*" (Malachi 3:2–3). In other words, people have to go through a process of refining before God will be real in their lives.

Effortless change

It would be ideal if the mind were perfectly clear and present in the moment, with no obstacles and blockages. To achieve that, the brain must change. Being part of the body, your brain has its own healing mechanisms. But old conditioning, once it gets established in your brain, becomes part of its neural networks. From your soul's perspective, these imprints are all subject to change. Moments of realization occur, and then however it is wired, the brain adapts. Unfortunately, current brain science accepts without question that brain changes are physical. Can we show that the brain is actually wireless? If we can, the way is open for awareness as the key to personal transformation.

That possibility took a huge leap forward when a team of Italian researchers in the 1980s was studying the brains of macaque monkeys. When a single neuron was monitored in a monkey's lower cortex, a region responsible for hand action, that neuron would fire when the animal reached for a piece of fruit, say a banana. In itself, this was a routine finding. Muscles move because the brain tells them to. But when the monkey saw another monkey reach for a banana, the same neuron fired again. In other words, *the act of seeing caused the first monkey's brain to fire as if it had performed the action itself.*

The concept of "mirror neurons" was born, meaning any neuron that imitates the action taking place in another, separate brain. The mirroring doesn't have to be between two like animals. A monkey watching a lab technician reaching for a banana will have its mirror neurons activated the same as if it were seeing another monkey perform the action. This response is not purely mechanical. A mirror neuron can tell the difference between an action it is interested in and one that it is indifferent to. For example, when a macaque monkey watches an experimenter put a piece of fruit in his mouth, a host of mirror neurons fire, but when the experimenter merely places the fruit in a bowl—an action the monkey shows little interest in—the mirror neurons barely fire.

This means that the brain's pathways do not have to be sculpted by direct physical experience. They can be shaped vicariously. Is that how we learn in the first place? It seems intuitive that a baby monkey, for example, learns to grab things by reaching out for them. But intuition is wrong in this case, because a baby monkey's brain doesn't have the neural pathways to perform the action for the first time. The purpose of mirror neurons is to build those pathways simply by looking—or, more precisely, by paying attention and being interested. Those words should sound familiar, because the Tibetan monks whose brains had neural networks for compassion built those networks the same way.

The brain doesn't even need instructions to make new pathways. Baby monkeys that are still nursing will watch their mothers eating solid food, and the mirror neurons inside their brains are activated as if they are eating solid food themselves. When weaning time comes, the brain is prepared. An unknown world becomes familiar simply by looking. Human learning may occur the same way, but no one knows yet. For ethical reasons, brain cells can't be wired for study in human infants, but by looking at eye movements, it appears that babies develop a mirroring system in the first year of life simply by paying attention to significant events around them.

Is this how you learn from the soul, too? We have one strong clue that it is. Think back to the phenomenon of *darshan*—the transmission of a blessing when someone is in the presence of a saint. Sages believe that merely setting eyes on a saint brings the blessing, and now we can see how: the devotee's brain is changed by the act of looking. "Blessing" is too mild a term, because in its highest form, known as *atman darshan*, there is a direct transmission from one soul (or *atman*) to another. It couldn't have occurred to anyone that mirror neurons were at work. The notion was unknown to me as a child visiting local saints. But the effects I felt—buoyancy, elation, inner peace—didn't require any understanding on my part. Someone else's soul had effortlessly changed my brain.

Why, then, can't my own soul do the same?

All the soul has to do is radiate its influence. If simply being close to a saint is enough, how much closer are you and I to our own souls? Higher consciousness is a field, like electricity or magnetism, and when a person comes into contact with that field, the brain mirrors it. The word *darshan* derives from the verb "to see," but your eyes don't have to be open; it is nearness to the field that causes the effect.

Going deeper, one finds that higher consciousness isn't static. A saint can transmit a specific energy, such as healing, and the target can be one person. Consider the passages in the New Testament where Jesus is implored to heal the sick. He is often reluctant, because he wants his listeners to go inside themselves to discover the Kingdom of Heaven—in essence, he's telling them that the field is part of themselves. External miracles pull attention in the wrong direction. When Jesus does happen to heal the lame, halt, and blind, he attributes the miracle to the one who was healed, not to himself.

Mark 10:46–52 offers a dramatic example, centering on a blind beggar sitting by the side of the road as Jesus walks by.

> *When he heard that it was Jesus of Nazareth, he began to shout out and say, "Jesus, Son of David, have mercy on me!" Many sternly ordered him to be quiet, but he cried out even more loudly, "Son of David, have mercy on me!" Jesus stood still and said, "Call him here." And they called the blind man, saying to him, "Take heart; get up, he is calling you." So throwing off his cloak, he sprang up and came to Jesus. Then Jesus said to him, "What do you want me to do for you?" The blind man said to him, "My teacher, let me see again." Jesus said to him, "Go; your*

*faith has made you well." Immediately he regained his sight
and followed him on the way.*

One is struck that the blind man seems more insistent than faithful, but in the tradition of *darshan*, the incident makes sense. Healing depends on connecting higher consciousness to lower, a perfect soul sending energy to an imperfect body. (Jesus' intervention wouldn't be needed, except as he says regretfully of his disciples, "The spirit is willing but the flesh is weak." In other words, their bodies are not perfectly attuned to the soul, while Jesus' is.) The body has no choice but to shift, just as a magnet has no choice but to point north. What could be more effortless?

Pauline's story

"Everyone who knows me says that I lead a charmed life," said Pauline, a professional woman who is now forty. "Some shake their heads and say it enviously, or with disbelief. But almost no one knows the truth. There's a reason everything goes right for me."

I raised my eyebrows. "Everything?"

Pauline nodded. "I haven't had a setback in twenty years. Things happen that look like problems to other people, but in the end they always turn out well. No matter what." She wasn't smug, or smiling as if she were keeping a mischievous secret. Pauline had something serious in mind.

"It all goes back to a very stressful time in my life. I was out of college but had no direction. At twenty-five I had landed in a civil service job that had nothing to offer except security. I dated, but there was no one serious. These sound like ordinary complaints, and they don't convey how terribly restless and dissatisfied I felt. I would wake up in the middle of the night gasping for breath, like somebody drowning.

"Nobody knew how I felt. What was there to say? Nobody could tell me what was really going on, at least not anyone I knew."

"Do you know now?" I asked.

Pauline nodded. "I was breaking up inside. No, that's too dramatic. I was reshuffling. The whole process must have been going on for a while, maybe since childhood; I was intensely religious at ten years old, dressing in black and retreating up into the attic to read the Bible. Anyway, I didn't know how to handle my restless state, which came to a head one Saturday afternoon.

"I was sitting by the window in an old armchair, my mind racing. I can't remember what my thoughts were about, but I do recall wondering if this is how people lose their minds."

"Did you feel crazy?" I asked.

She shook her head. "That's the funny thing. I wasn't agitated emotionally. A strange kind of calm had settled over me. It was like watching somebody else's mind racing faster and faster. Suddenly it all stopped. I looked outside at the bright summer sun, and I knew. *Everything you want is coming to you. There's nothing to do.* Just like that. I couldn't believe it."

"Did you hear a voice in your head?" I asked.

"No. But it felt as if somebody was communicating with me. God? My higher self? I wouldn't want to put a name to that inner voice, but my body became very relaxed. I thought I was going to cry, but instead I gave an enormous sigh. A huge burden was lifted that I didn't even know I was carrying."

"In one epiphany you got a charmed life?" I said.

"Yes." Pauline was unblinking.

"Right away?"

"Not quite. At first I went around in a state of euphoria. I had complete trust in what the voice told me. I saw everything through rose-colored glasses. You see, I had no fear anymore. People don't realize it, but fear is always lurking somewhere in the background, like termites in the woodwork. When it's gone, the whole world brightens up.

"That phase lasted only a few weeks. I came down off my high. I was more myself again. You'd think that was the end of it. But in fact the change was real. Bad things stopped happening to me. I started making choices that were right. My existence was no longer full of crises and drama. Other people began to notice that I was leading a charmed life."

One could see from Pauline's calm certainty that she didn't care if anyone believed her. I congratulated her, we chatted awhile longer about the good things that kept happening to her, and then she left. I have rarely met anyone who is a better example of the soul's field effect. The voice she heard didn't come from outside herself. We could say that she heard her soul's voice, but the soul is silent. Rather, she heard her own mind putting into words a shift in consciousness. Such shifts are unpredictable; you never know beforehand that you are going to take a quantum leap (although going through a period of turbulence, as Pauline did, is quite common). There are many kinds of epiphanies, and it is mistaken to categorize them all as religious. What all epiphanies do have in common, however, is that awareness expands beyond its normal boundaries.

I would call this an epiphany about surrender. Imagine that you are caught between two forces. One, the force of conditioning, pulls you toward a life full of effort and struggle. The other, the force of the soul, pulls you toward a life that is effortless. The contest appears to be grossly unfair, because the first force has a huge alliance behind it. Everyone you know accepts that life is difficult, and therefore society demands that you go along, not only in word and deed, but even in the thoughts that run through your head. For your thoughts are not your own. You have assimilated a hundred voices from the wider environment—family, friends, mass media, society in general—and now they speak to you from inside your own mind.

Compared with this massive alliance, the soul has no visible power. It has no voice in your head. It is too intimate for other people to explain to you. We have seen that awareness can move energy, but the soul's awareness is so refined that the energy it moves is incredibly subtle. With so much going against it, how does the soul exert any force at all? The answer is surprisingly simple. Your soul is you. Outside forces exert constant pressure, and in the short run, your soul's signals will be blocked out. But in the end you can't ignore yourself. By being ever-present, your soul can wait as long as it takes.

You can perform a simple experiment to prove this to yourself. Consider another ever-present thing: breathing. You spend hours ignoring your breath. It proceeds without cessation, never drawing attention to itself. Now sit still and try to ignore your breathing. Deliberately make an effort to shut it out. You can't. Once your attention has been drawn to your breathing, a change has occurred. Eventually, of course, your mind will wander. You will lapse back into forgetfulness of your breath. But that makes no difference to it. Like the soul, your breath can afford to wait, since it is ever-present as long as your are alive.

In Pauline's case, what really happened wasn't an epiphany in the ordinary sense. God on high didn't suddenly notice her and send a special telegram. Rather, she noticed her soul the same way a person notices his breathing. In itself, that's not a unique occurrence. Each of us has passing moments when we slip inadvertently into a higher state of consciousness. The trick is to keep your mind from wandering away again. Pauline achieved something rare: she noticed her soul and then didn't take her attention off it. The soul's presence remained with her, which is why her life became "charmed."

This may seem like a special case, but the general principle holds true for everyone. If you can bring your attention to the level of the soul, struggle ceases. The first thing to change is your perspective, but there are changes in the way that life treats you as well. These are more mysterious. Our society doesn't accept that the soul—invisible, eternal, detached, unmoving, and immortal—has the power to transform the stubborn world of concrete objects and material events. Yet for life to become easier, the soul must have that power. There are levels of mystery yet to explore.

In Your Life: Creating Your Own Epiphany

It's unfortunate that the word *epiphany* is limited to a religious context. People assume that epiphanies are about God and occur only to saints. An epiphany is really a mini-breakthrough. One piece of conditioning is shattered. Instead of being the victim of a rigid belief, you feel released. What causes such a mini-breakthrough? You have to shift your attention to the soul, because that is the aspect of yourself that is not conditioned. The soul represents higher awareness in that sense—it is free from all conditioning. Or, to put it most simply, the soul never says no. Anything is possible. Whatever can be imagined comes true. If you can keep your attention on your soul, you will experience an epiphany every day. Instead of *no*, you will experience unlimited *yes*.

To get beyond the power of *no* is crucially important. *No* is very convincing. People reject all kinds of experiences because they believe it's right to reject. They oppose because they can't bring themselves not to. The spell of *no* holds them so strongly that little else matters. Some concrete examples will help here, then we will see how each one can be reversed.

Getting Past *No*

You must break the spell when your mind:

- tells you that people don't change
- keeps you trapped in rigid habits
- traps the mind in obsessive thoughts
- creates cravings that cannot be appeased
- puts up fear as a threat if you try to break free
- forbids you to have certain thoughts
- makes natural urges seem illicit or dangerous

It takes mini-breakthroughs to get past the power of no because there is so much negativity to overcome in so many areas. But in each area the same principle holds: to make life easier, you need to stop doing whatever it is that you're doing. I know this sounds terribly general, but in reality if you were doing the right thing, you would be in contact with your soul already, and you life would be unfolding, day by day, on the principle of *yes*. So you have to stop what you're doing and shake things up.

Now let's look at the specific areas where the power of no needs to be dislodged.

Negative Belief #1: People don't change. This familiar assertion seems reasonable in moments of discouragement and frustration, but if you look more closely, it has the effect of shutting down change in yourself. In essence, if other people can't or won't change, we're fated to live in the status quo. When you assume nobody is going to change, you have closed the box and locked them in. At the same time, you get locked in, too. It's easy to miss that implication, because in our heart of hearts, we secretly believe that *we* can change; it's only other people who can't. In reality, they feel the same about you, and so a system of mutual discouragement is set up. In short order, anyone who stands up and says "we need to change" is bucking the status quo. And anyone who breaks away and actually does change is viewed with suspicion, or with outright hostility.

From your soul's perspective, however, none of this is real. It's obvious that people constantly change. We hunger for news; we inflame daily life into crises, large and small. Our moods shift, as does every cell in our bodies. To say that people don't change is arbitrary, a point of view that seems safe. It's a form of resignation, of giving in to the inevitable. You must stop reinforcing the power of no if you want to reach your soul.

- See yourself as changing all the time.
- Encourage change in others.
- When you hear yourself uttering a fixed opinion, stop.
- When someone offers a counter-opinion, don't resist.
- Argue from the opposite side every once in a while.
- Don't stamp out the fragile beginnings of change, either in yourself or in others.

- Stop being absolute. Let your attitude be more flexible and provisional.
- Don't take pride in being right.
- When you have an impulse to grow and evolve, follow it without regard for the opinions of others.

Negative Belief #2: Habits keep us trapped. Everyone knows what it means to be caught up in habitual behavior. Life's everyday struggle is dominated by our inability to think and behave in a new way. Habits keep married couples locked in the same argument for years. It makes us plop down on the couch rather than work for change. It reinforces bad diets and lack of exercise. In general, habit makes inertia easier than change. Here the force of no is fairly obvious—or is it? If you look at it without negative judgments, a habit is nothing more than a useful shortcut, an automatic pathway imprinted in the brain. A skilled pianist has imprinted the habit of moving his fingers a certain way; he wouldn't want to reinvent his technique every time he sat down at the keyboard. A short-order cook who can turn out six omelets at a time relies on the fact that his brain is imprinted with a set of automatic motions precisely timed.

From your soul's perspective, a habit is just a choice that is ingrained for practical purposes. There's no issue of good and bad, right or wrong. You always have the choice to erase the imprint and create a new one. A pianist who takes up the violin isn't hampered by the imprinted way his fingers used to move. A short-order cook who goes home to make one omelet instead of six isn't compelled to work at lightning speed. What keeps us trapped is the spell of no. In the grip of that spell, we find reasons to keep being stuck in habitual thinking and behaviors when they no longer serve us. We voluntarily renounce the power to change, while at the same time blaming our bad habits, as if they had an independent will (currently it's fashionable to blame the brain, as if its imprints are permanent and all-powerful). To break out of any habit, you need to reclaim your power to choose.

- Don't fight against a bad habit. Look at it objectively, as if another person had the habit.
- Ask yourself why you have chosen your habit.
- Examine what benefit you are getting, usually at a hidden level.
- Be honest about your choice. Instead of saying, "This is just how I am," admit that you have chosen inertia over change because change frightens or threatens you.
- If you feel victimized by a bad habit, ask yourself why you need to be a victim. Is it an easy way to keep from taking responsibility?
- Find a reason to adopt a good habit in place of the bad one; make your reason convincing, and keep repeating it to yourself whenever the old habit arises.

Your aim is to break the spell that says you have no choices. You always have choices.

Negative Belief #3: Obsessive thoughts are in control. Most people don't think they are obsessive. They identify obsessions with mental disorders, when in fact an obsessive-compulsive disorder is just an extreme variation on a universal condition. Obsessions are yet another way that the power of no removes your ability to choose. At any given moment you might obsess about keeping safe, avoiding germs, getting angry in traffic, spending money, disciplining your children, defeating terrorism—the possibilities are endless and ever-changing. You can't assume that a thought becomes an obsession only if it's immoral, wrong, or irrational. One can obsess about things that society approves of and rewards. We all know people who obsess about winning, or getting back at those who wronged them, or money, or ambition. By definition, an obsessive thought is one that's stronger than you are. That's where the power of no does its damage.

From the soul's perspective, thinking is an expression of freedom.

The mind isn't compelled to prefer one thought over another. Much less is the mind a machine programmed to repeat the same message over and over. What keeps us trapped in repetition is the belief that "I *must* think this way." Other alternatives are closed off by fear, prejudice, self-interest, and guilt. To break out of obsessive thinking, you must examine this deeper level where "I must" holds sway.

- Don't struggle against thoughts that keep repeating themselves.
- When people tell you that you keep doing the same thing, believe them.
- Don't accept that always winning, always being out for number one, or always doing *anything* is productive.
- Don't pride yourself on consistency for consistency's sake.
- If you feel trapped by an obsession, ask yourself what you're afraid of. Repetition is a mask for anxiety.
- Stop rationalizing. Put your attention on how your thoughts feel, not on what they say.
- Be honest about the frustration you feel with having the same idea over and over.
- Don't defend your prejudices.
- Take active steps to reduce stress, which is a major cause of obsessions. Under stress, the mind keeps repeating the same thing because it isn't relaxed or open enough to find an alternative.
- Through meditation, seek the level of your mind that isn't obsessed, that has no fixed ideas.

Negative Belief #4: Cravings can never be appeased. When cravings keep returning, they force you either to give in or resist (the futility of this struggle was touched on earlier). The power of no insists that you have no other alternative. Once again, a repetitive pattern imprinted in the brain overrides free choice. Your craving takes on a life of its own, and if taken to extremes, it becomes an addiction. The difference has to do with just how limited you become. Someone who craves chocolate can't resist eating some, but if addicted, they would eat nothing else. Even in its milder forms, however, craving can make you feel that you have no other choice.

From your soul's perspective, a craving is another example of a shortcut imprinted in the brain. The person who always eats chocolate has made an implicit choice that chocolate is the best kind of sweet, and therefore, instead of his being bothered every time to consider a variety of sweets, he chooses chocolate automatically. But setting your mind on autopilot doesn't mean that you can't change it. The option to reset your reactions always exists. Under the spell of no, you willingly gave up that option, but anything you give up you can also reclaim.

- When a craving arises, don't make it an either/or choice.
- Instead of either giving in or resisting, do one of the following: walk away, postpone your choice, find a distraction, pause and watch yourself, or substitute another pleasure.
- Don't think of defeating your craving. Think instead that you are gradually erasing an imprint.
- When you feel discouraged for giving in, be with your feelings instead of pushing them away.
- Realize why appeasing a craving never works: you can never get enough of what you didn't want in the first place.
- Find out what you really want, whether it's love, comfort, approval, or security. These are the basic needs that cravings try to substitute for.
- Pursue your real need. If you do, the craving will automatically lose its grip and in time will vanish.
- If for any reason you can turn away from your old craving, seize that moment, even if your craving soon returns. Every small victory imprints the brain in a new pattern. Don't see this as a temporary victory—see it as a sign that you can find the switch that turns your craving off.

Negative Belief #5: Fear keeps you from being free. The power of no
uses fear as its enforcer. Like a hired gun, it holds a threat that is merciless
and indifferent. Under the spell of no, the mind finds any and every reason to be afraid. The simplest things become objects of anxiety. The most
unlikely risks loom as dangers that can befall you at any moment. When
you find yourself in a defensive posture, you have denied yourself the
most basic freedom, which is to be safe in the world. It's not the external
threat that creates this situation. We project our fixed beliefs onto every
situation, so feeling safe or unsafe becomes a personal decision.

From the soul's perspective, you are always safe. The universe
cherishes your existence. Nature is designed to uphold your well-
being. If you find yourself under threat, it can be quite realistic to
assess the danger and escape it. But if you are paralyzed by anxiety, the
threat becomes inescapable. Someone with a fear of heights, for
example, finds it impossible to climb a stepladder. The danger of
falling doesn't prevent other people from climbing the ladder, because
they are free to assess that the risk is small. But a phobia takes away the
freedom to assess danger realistically; fear acquires absolute power, the
power of no. To get beyond a phobia, you must call its bluff and
reassert that you are safe.

- Don't fight your fears when you are actually afraid.
- When you feel calm and safe, call your fear to mind so that it
  can be examined.
- Fear is convincing, but that doesn't make it right. Make sure
  you see this distinction.
- Anxiety tends to obsess about reasons to be afraid, stoking its
  own fire. Don't be fooled by repetition. A situation doesn't
  become more dangerous just because you keep thinking it is.
- Separate the energy of fear from the content of your experience. Instead of worrying about the thing that makes you
  anxious, go directly to the feeling of anxiety and move the
  energy as you would any other, through physical release, toning, meditation, and other techniques.

- Realize that you are not basically afraid. Fear is a passing emotion that can be released.
- Know that you have a choice to either hold on to fear or let it go. If you feel anxious, take immediate steps to let go. Don't dwell on fear or try to reason with it.
- Avoid blaming yourself. Fear is universal. It is felt by the bravest, strongest people. To be afraid doesn't mean you are weak. It means you haven't yet let go.
- Be patient with yourself. Fear and anxiety are the biggest obstacles for everyone. Be thankful and congratulate yourself every time you overcome fear.
- Don't consider it a defeat if fear returns. The time will soon come when you can sit calmly and move the energy of fear. Ultimately you are the one in control.

Negative Belief #6: "Bad" thoughts are forbidden and dangerous.
People expend a lot of subtle energy in pushing down thoughts they don't want to face. Denial and repression seem appealing as short-term solutions. What you don't think about may go away. But there's a sticky quality to bad thoughts—which are any thoughts that make you feel guilty, ashamed, humiliated, or distressed. And denial only makes the pain worse over time. Delay also makes it harder to release old, stuck energies when you finally decide that they must be confronted.

If you choose to push bad thoughts out of sight, that's your decision. The danger comes when you begin to believe that certain thoughts are forbidden as if by a law of outside force. When that happens, the power of no has convinced you that your own mind is your enemy. Many people, including trained psychotherapists, are threatened by the "shadow," a name given to the forbidden zone of the mind where dangerous urges lurk. Under the spell of no, you fear your shadow and believe that you should never go near it.

From the soul's perspective, the mind has no boundaries. If you feel that it is forbidden to look at your rage, fear, jealousy, desperation, and feelings of vengeance, you are resorting to a false sense of self. Specifically, you are dividing yourself into good and bad impulses. The paradox is that your good side can never ultimately win, because the bad side will constantly fight to be released. An inner struggle ensues. You wind up living in a state of underground warfare. Instead of trying to be good all the time, try to win your freedom. When the mind is free, thoughts come and go spontaneously. Whether good or bad, you don't hold on to them. As long as the mind is allowed to flow, no thought is dangerous, and therefore nothing is forbidden.

- See the difference between having a "bad" thought and acting on it.
- Don't identify with your thoughts. They aren't you; they are passing events in the mind.
- Resist the urge to demonize. Judgment makes illicit impulses stick around.
- Learn the value of acceptance.
- Don't condemn others for their thoughts.
- Don't set up a false ideal of yourself. See clearly that every kind of thought, mood, and sensation exists in your makeup.
- Celebrate the diversity of your mind. A mind that is free to think any way it wants should be appreciated, not suppressed.
- If you were taught that God will hate you for sinful thoughts, try to detach yourself from this perspective. Holding a judgmental God responsible for your own self-judgment is a delusion.
- Don't fixate on being right all the time. Being right is just a disguise for making other people wrong. In the shadows, you secretly fear that something is wrong with you, which is why you fight so hard to appear infallible—you think it makes you good.

- When you are tempted to control your mind, stand back and realize that the task is impossible to begin with. Even the most disciplined mind has a way of breaking out of its chains.

Negative Belief #7: Natural urges are illicit or dangerous. Since there is no such thing as an artificial urge, all urges are natural. They arise from either a desire or a need. When the mind intervenes, however, any urge can become a danger. Eating a candy bar feels dangerous if you are obsessed with your weight. Loving somebody feels dangerous if you fear rejection. There is a tangled dance between what we feel and what we think we should feel, and everyone is caught up in the dance, which is why disputes over social values can lead to violence. People have a lot at stake in judging right from wrong, and invoking God or higher morality to justify their own sense of guilt and shame. The power of no insists that right and wrong are absolutes. Under its spell, you become afraid of what you actually feel. Unable to assess your feelings in a positive light, you allow them to become distorted. As a result, more and more energy is spent defending white against black, without regard for the fact that violence even in the defense of right is wrong.

From your soul's perspective, all urges are based on legitimate needs. When the need is seen and fulfilled, the urge fades away, just as hunger fades once you eat. However, when a need is denied or judged against, it has no choice but to become more insistent. Urges build up, pushing against the resistance that is trying to hold them down. At a certain point this war between urge and resistance becomes so strident that you lose sight of the original need.

When someone is pulled toward illicit sexual urges, for example, it is all but certain that a simple need—for love, gratification, self-worth, or acceptance—has become deeply buried. All that's visible is the illicit urge and the war it wages with shame and guilt. If the illicit urge is rage and hostility, the underlying need is almost always the need to be safe and unafraid. So the ultimate issue isn't whether you can win the battle against our "bad" urges, but whether you can find the need that fuels them. When you can satisfy a basic need, impulse control is no longer a problem.

Stop seeing this as a matter of self-control. Every kind of urge comes and goes in everyone.

- Be willing to stop judging against yourself. Bad urges don't make you a bad person.
- Know that neither side will ever win an internal war.
- Don't make this a test of willpower. Giving in to an urge isn't proof that you need to discipline yourself even more.
- Permissiveness isn't a viable solution, any more than is its opposite, rigid self-discipline. Acting on your urges serves only as a temporary release of energy, like opening a steam gasket. There will always be more steam.
- Your personal demons will get worse if you keep being ashamed of them.
- Guilt is a perception, and all perceptions are open to change. You can't instantly change guilt to approval, but you can see guilt as negotiable. When you remove the underlying energy that forces you to be guilty, a new perception can flower.
- Realize that your soul never judges you. With that in mind, your aim is to live from the level of the soul. That is the final answer to the war between good and bad.

Breakthrough #2

Love Awakens the Soul

A breakthrough at the soul level expands love, but it also brings challenges. The soul takes God's infinite love and steps it down to human scale. How much intensity of love you can receive depends on many things. Most people dream of more love in their lives, yet in reality the amount they have right now is what they have adapted to. There's also the issue of how acceptable it is to show intense love. Not everyone would be comfortable if you suddenly confronted them with an onrush of unconditional love. They would wonder if this new kind of love could be trusted. In their heart of hearts they would worry that they didn't deserve such open, complete love.

Many people have made momentary contact with the soul's more intense, purer love. When they do, there's a wonderful sense of awakening. Love awakens the soul. This happens because like is attracted to like. The soul isn't passive. It vibrates in sympathy with you anytime you try to free yourself from limitations. There's a similar sense of expansion and liberation when you experience beauty or truth. You are freeing up soul energy and letting it flow. The electricity in your house doesn't provide light and heat until you flick a switch. Something very similar happens when you awaken the soul's energy.

People experience a surge of the soul's energy without knowing exactly how they did it. Without warning they glimpse unconditional love or feel God's presence. There's a sense of being blissful and unbounded. It suddenly feels real to go beyond all boundaries. Why, then, does everyday life draw them back down again? These privileged journeys into expanded awareness are almost always brief—a matter of moments, perhaps a few days, and rarely more than a few months.

Year after year the brain has adapted to a way of life in which it is normal to be much less than loving and joyful. Since you can't force yourself to embrace something new, what will do it? The answer, I believe, is desire. The desire to love and be loved constantly urges each person forward. When that desire is most alive, we seek the most from life. When that desire flickers out, life becomes static.

Countless people prefer to exist without love because they are too afraid to risk whatever comfort they have; others have failed in love and feel wounded, or have grown bored with someone they once loved. For all these people, love has come to a stop, which means that an aspect of the soul is numb. To tell someone in that condition that love is infinite may be inspiring, but the inspiration is empty unless they can experience not infinite love, but the next step. And the next step is always the same: to awaken the soul. Because everyone is different, there's no cut-and-dried method to achieve this. It may work to tell a lonely person to get out of the house and meet new people, go on a date, or join an Internet service that matches couples up. And it may not work at all.

The secret of desire

Why is love like water to one thirsty soul and yet rejected by another? I'm reminded of a poignant story told to me by a woman from the Southwest who retired from a lucrative media job to become a builder. She chose to buy land in the most dilapidated section of the barrio, where she intended to renovate a group of adobe houses. "It was a hard choice to be a builder in those surroundings," she recalls. "I hired local workmen, but there was a lot of theft from the site. Many of the men were out of work and resented having a woman boss. Every day the kids on the block would gather at the curb to stare at me framing out a roof or plastering a wall. None of them had ever seen a new house being built, I imagine.

"Two kids caught my eye. Antonio was older than the others, maybe fifteen. He had a drug history and a string of arrests. But one day I came to the site and found a mural of the Virgin Mary painted on a wall. When I asked around, Antonio confessed that he had done it. So I made a secret pact with him. I bought him the materials that local painters used to make traditional *retablos*, holy pictures painted on tin. He eagerly went to work, and it wasn't long before he had an active little business going. Nobody talked about what I'd done for him, but they knew.

"The other kid was a little girl, Carla, who was eight or nine, very bright and very curious. We got to be friends, and I met her mother. I was so touched by their sweetness, people who had almost nothing, that I went to the best private school in town and got the principal to agree to admit Carla on a full scholarship.

"I took time off and helped her mother send her off that first morning, and then I went back to work. Around one o'clock I looked over and saw Carla where she always was, standing with the other kids watching the workmen. She was no longer in her school dress. I felt very upset and ran down the street to the trailer where the family lived.

"I asked the mother what had gone wrong. Did Carla misbehave? Did the other kids pick on her? She looked away, not wanting to meet my eyes. 'I went back at noon and took Carla home,' she said. 'You tried to do a nice thing, but she doesn't belong there. She'd never fit in.' I tried not to get angry. I coaxed and cajoled, but the mother was firm, and her little girl never went back."

The moral of this story is that love and desire must match. The spiritual path unfolds when you follow your heart's desire. Inside everyone is a place that is intimate, alive, and full of yearning. It doesn't focus on God, or salvation, or unconditional love. It focuses on the next thing it desires. If that next thing is fulfilled, there will be another next thing, and then another, and on and on. Religious traditions miss this very pragmatic point. They offer the final, glorious reward to people who can't figure out how to get the next small reward. No religion can dictate from the outside. Only you are in touch with the living impulse of desire that wants to move ahead.

But what if the next thing you want to do is eat chocolate cake?

What if your deepest hunger is for a second house or a third wife? The soul doesn't judge your desires. It works with who you are and where you are now. The trick is to turn the path of desire, which for most people is focused on worldly things, and redirect it to a higher plane.

The problem of boundaries

As much as you may love chocolate cake or a second house, there's a limit to the joy that material things bring. The great disadvantage to desire is that repetition kills joy. Couples face this problem in marriage, because daily life with another person, however much you love that person, involves a great deal of repetition. The standard advice is to add spice by doing something new. Surprise your husband with new lingerie. Surprise your wife with a vacation in Bermuda. This advice may work in the short run, but it's only a temporary diversion. There's a deeper answer based on the soul.

As your soul sees it, desire has no interest in repetition. It wants to go deeper. It wants more intensity, more meaning, more expansion. What keeps a marriage alive is that you see more to love in your partner; the possibilities grow over time. Intimacy with another person is an incredible discovery, for which there is no substitute. When you find such intimacy, you naturally want more—you want it to grow closer. On the other hand, desire that doesn't go deeper, which circles around repeating the same pattern over and over, has somehow been diverted from its natural course.

If this description brings images to mind of a dog chasing its tail, or racing cars endlessly marking laps on the track, you have grasped the point perfectly. Desire that pursues its object while never gaining ground is stuck. A boundary acts like an invisible fence or a line that is not supposed to be crossed. Why do we put boundaries around our desires? First, to keep out uncomfortable experiences. Think of the times you've passed a panhandler or beggar on the street—or a Santa ringing a bell for charity at Christmas, for that matter. If you decide to freeze out their pleas, you put up an invisible barrier. Because it is psychological, a boundary can have emotional implications for the person who sets it in place. Imagine yourself as the panhandler instead. When you say "Spare change?" some people will simply ignore you; others will hurry their steps out of guilt; many more will be irritated or angry; a few might ironically toss you a penny or act deeply offended.

The second reason for putting up a boundary is to protect your comfort zone. Inside this zone you feel satisfied. You also feel safe and protected. There are many kinds of comfort zones. For every person who feels safe only when he or she is alone, there's another who feels safe only when other people are around. But whatever kind of zone you have created, you are making it much harder to allow change into your life. When I was a medical intern rotating through various departments of the hospital, I learned some acute lessons about why people don't change. One of my most vivid memories from a veterans hospital outside Boston was of leaning out the window of the cafeteria, watching patients down below.

Each patient was wheeled to the front door of the hospital, at which point he got up and walked away. A happy sight, you would think. But one day I saw a lung cancer patient under my care cross the street and enter a drugstore. Two minutes later he came out with a carton of cigarettes under his arm. He had already ripped open a pack and lit up the first smoke. When I pointed this out to a second-year oncology resident, he shrugged and told me that if he looked out the window, he'd see half of his patients doing the same thing. He had learned not to look.

This was thirty years ago, and fortunately the tide has turned against smoking. But the deeper point is that people will go a long way to protect their comfort zones and to fence out painful reality. Another memory from those days, this one from a time when I was on psychiatric rotation: a woman came in for evaluation, and as I was doing her workup, she revealed that she had four young children at home and a husband who had lost his job and started to drink. She was diabetic and many pounds overweight. I felt overwhelmed at what her life must be like, but when I asked her why she had come to the clinic, she said, "I have a feeling I'm depressed, but I can't figure out why."

Back then I assumed that offering kindness, sympathy, and caring would nourish everyone—I underestimated how protective boundaries really are, thinking they would be easy to tear down. Boundaries are made of frozen awareness, which is very elusive to understand. I had a very warm-hearted mentor on my psych rotation who was considered the most empathetic doctor in the hospital. He could get people to open up who seemed frozen and out of reach. He himself was a delightfully open, carefree person, and he used his natural charm to disarm frightened patients.

But he also had deep understanding of why these people were unreachable. It's one thing to feel unloved, he said, but for some, "I am unlovable" is such a deeply ingrained belief that it feels like part of who they are. So when you expose them to love and caring, they flee. Why shouldn't they? You are threatening to take away part of their identity, which would be threatening to anyone. Try going home next Christmas or Thanksgiving and being kind to the relative who bothers you the most. When you radiate love where once you radiated dislike, their response will probably be suspicion, and if you persist, they may become anxious or angry.

In short, our boundaries are part of our identities. The soul can change that identity, and the process begins by negotiating with your boundaries. You know, in your heart of hearts, that you aren't truly safe, protected, or fulfilled. If you want those things to be real, several new assumptions come into play:

- You are not so afraid of risk.
- You don't have to be right all the time.
- You trust that love is meant for you.
- You welcome the opportunity to expand.
- You see abundance as natural to life.
- You don't expect anything.

These are powerful beliefs, and they all melt boundaries. Let's take a closer look at how they work.

You are not so afraid of risk. Taking a risk is the same as stepping outside your boundary. We all want to be free, but anxiety holds us back. Every mother knows the look a toddler wears when it first tries to walk—it's a mixture of curiosity, intention, anxiety, and open-eyed wonder. "What am I doing? I know I want to try this, but it feels wild." That's the look of a risk-taker. It expresses the mixed feelings that are inescapable when you abandon what you know for what you don't. Boundaries try to convince us that risks are too dangerous. In truth, risk-taking is desire coaxing you to reach for something new.

People who avoid all risks are making a devil's bargain. In exchange for limited fulfillment, they gain safety. But that safety is an illusion. The reality is that they are stuck, immobile. Think of an agoraphobe, someone who is afraid to go outdoors or into large open spaces. Staying at home feels safe at first, because the outside has been walled off. But as time passes, even the safety of being in the house starts to lose its effect. Now the agoraphobic sufferer finds himself feeling comfortable in only one room, and then a smaller room, until only the smallest room in the house brings any feeling of security. Why does the phobia progress this way? Because the desire to be outside can't be stifled, and as it builds up, the phobia counters by creating tighter and tighter boundaries. Learning that risks are positive, that they allow you to grow, is an important step.

You don't have to be right all the time. Being inside a limiting boundary is like being the ruler of a small island. You are in control, and the essence of control is always being right. I once met a strong-minded man, an executive in a large corporation, who had the annoying habit of contradicting everyone who tried to talk to him. His automatic reaction to any statement, no matter how obvious or innocuous, was "That's not true" (or "There's another way of looking at this," "I'm not sure about that," or "That's a weak argument," etc.). Apparently he was unaware that he did this. He had just gotten into the habit of making everyone else wrong so that he could always be right. An associate of his asked me to assess what was going on. I sat and listened while this man spent an hour contradicting each person he came into contact with. I decided to try the direct approach and pointed out that he had said "That's not true" at least twice a minute all morning. Without the slightest hesitation he turned to me and said, "That's not true."

Notice how much is contained in those few words. "That's not true" allows someone to shut out anyone who disagrees, and to put up a warning sign that reads, "Keep out. My mind is already closed." Boundaries, it turns out, serve very complicated purposes; they can't be defined purely as psychological defenses. In this case, learning that you don't have to be right means learning to trust, because the basic need expressed is for control. The boundary is only strengthened if you challenge it; trying to prove to a control personality that he is wrong is futile. Instead, you must show, over and over, that your love can be trusted.

If this boundary is your own, the best approach is to trust someone else in a small way every day. That means not telling them in advance how to do things, not nitpicking and indulging in perfectionism, not contradicting and insisting that only you know what's right. Reversing our habit of being right will feel uncomfortable— that's only natural. But for every time that your trust is rewarded, you will have one reason fewer to put up your old wall.

You trust that love is meant for you. Many kinds of boundaries hide self-judgment. People who reject intimacy feel that they don't deserve love. They fear exposure, not wanting other people to see how unlovable they are. Putting up a boundary also allows them not to look at why they feel they don't deserve love. (In place of love, you can substitute respect, admiration, acceptance, appreciation—these are all offshoots of love.) The most fortunate among us have been loved since birth. But that is rare. Most people have experienced a combination of love and rejection, even when very young. They have been exposed to negative situations in which their worthiness remains a question.

The only cure for this doubt is to be loved, and that won't happen if you shut yourself off. Unfortunately, the more you feel you don't deserve love, the more you isolate yourself, and then the certainty that you don't deserve love grows stronger. In essence, you can only attract and hold on to as much love as you feel for yourself. One sees evidence for this when a woman says, "I keep dating the same man over and over," or "I only meet men who wind up rejecting me." In the case of men, the complaint is the same, but with gender variations: "I meet a lot of women, but nobody I'd marry," or "I love women, but I don't want to be pressured to settle down." Society provides all kinds of ready-made responses behind which a person can hide from his or her own self-judgment.

This limiting boundary can be taken down by trusting that you are lovable, not completely (that would be asking too much), but enough to remain on the outer edge of your comfort zone. You can help a needy child, work for the poor, tutor a high-school dropout— these are acts of love that bring rewards just as big as going on a date, and usually more. As love comes to you, it will become part of your identity. Love wants to grow. You only need to plant the seed.

You welcome the opportunity to expand. People who live behind boundaries are suspicious of expanding. Human beings are unique in that expansion for us happens in awareness. For example, it's expansive to share and give. But the matter is complicated: the physical act of giving isn't sufficient. It's possible to give away millions while still being greedy and selfish at heart. There seems to be an innate mechanism that makes it almost physically necessary for some people to contract, withdraw, and hide. A recent social science experiment took a group of people and showed them a series of slides depicting gruesome events, such as war and automobile accidents. Each person was monitored to measure his or her response, using blood pressure, heart rate, and galvanic skin response. Everyone in the group found it stressful to look at the harrowing photos. But at a certain point some subjects became inured to what they were seeing. Their stress response tapered off, while for other subjects it didn't—they were just as upset by the last horrible sight as they were by the first. On the surface this experiment showed how quickly some of us build barriers against experiences that we find fearful. Another result turned out to be counterintuitive, however.

The people taking part had been asked beforehand to state their political preferences. As it turned out, those who labeled themselves liberal were the ones who quickly overcame their initial shock and got used to the gruesome pictures. Those who identified themselves as conservative were the ones who remained distressed. The experimenters struggled to explain this result, because the stereotype of bleeding-heart liberals would lead one to assume that they would be the most sensitive. But perhaps it takes a strong ability to accept the existence of pain and suffering in order to try to fix it, whereas people who remain shocked by pain and suffering only want to stop seeing it. You have to be comfortable with painful reality before you can actually help to do something about it.

The same applies to helping ourselves. It takes willingnes to face the darkness before the light can come in. Your soul treats your boundaries with utmost care. It never demands healing. It never crashes through, even with love. Here, I think the mind leads the emotions. Expansion happens on its own, but first your mind must give permission. Contraction is always based upon fear, and fear's grip is entirely emotional. Like a parent who coaxes a timid child into the water, you can negotiate with your fearful, contracted self. It takes skill.

The key step is to realize that even the tightest, most constricted part of yourself wants to be free. With that in mind, you ask yourself, "What do I want?" The answer doesn't have to be grand. You don't have to want total fulfillment, joy, and love. Find a feasible desire. The next thing that brings you joy, whatever it is, brings you closer to your soul. It may be mixed with discomfort, but if you can give yourself a truly expansive experience, your need to contract will begin to diminish. The more joy you are open to receiving, the less you'll need to have any boundaries at all.

You see abundance as natural to life. If you believe in scarcity, you cannot help but live in fear. Most of us consider our jobs, houses, bank accounts, and possessions defenses against scarcity. But inner lack is the real threat. Your body is an obvious example of Nature's abundance. Hundreds of billions of cells are provided for. Your blood surges through your arteries like a tidal wave. Likewise, your soul is a reservoir for infinite energy, creativity, and intelligence. It can't possibly run dry. This means little, however, if you believe that you are living in scarcity.

When that belief takes hold, it takes enormous struggle just to squeeze enough out of life to survive. This belief is common, ironically enough, among very wealthy people. Their riches keep them satiated externally while on the inside they feel famished. Hence they crave more and more of what didn't satisfy them in the first place.

There is a huge discrepancy, then, between what the soul is providing and what we receive. I find that when someone feels poor inside, the following exercise is very helpful. Take a piece of paper and write the word *Abundance,* then draw a circle around it. Now write five words around the circle, each one standing for an area that would make your life feel more abundant. (When I do this exercise with people, I ask them not to write material things like money, houses, or possessions. Career, work, and success are good substitutes, because they have an inner meaning.) Let's say the five words you wrote were:

Peace
Fun
Compassion
Well-being
Family

One man actually listed these five things. For him, life would be abundant if all of these areas were more fulfilled. Now, taking each item in turn, write down three things you can do, starting today, to make these areas more fulfilling. Here's a sample of what this man wrote:

> **Fun:** Spend more time outdoors.
>
> Play games with the kids.
>
> Learn to have fun again.
>
> **Compassion:** Give to the homeless guy on the block.
>
> Offer help to my depressed co-worker.
>
> Volunteer at local animal shelter.
>
> **Family:** Tell my wife more often that I love her.
>
> Sit at the dinner table and talk about how everyone is doing.
>
> Pay attention to signs of sadness and unhappiness.

It's not enough to yearn for more in your life. Your desire must be specific; it must point from where you are to where you want to be. Such a desire isn't chaotic or out of control. Rather, it exerts gentle pressure for change.

You don't expect anything. Nothing creates more unhappiness than failed expectations. The job promotion that doesn't come through, the proposal of marriage that is postponed one more time, the image of an ideal family that never materializes. Expectations are an attempt to control the future. An expectation says, "I won't be happy unless *x* happens." Here we must be careful, however. Having no expectations is a familiar way of saying that life is empty and without hope. That is not the goal. Instead, it's a kind of openness in which anything can happen and be welcomed.

Recently I had a vivid experience of this. A book tour had taken me to the tenth city in as many days. To survive the grind of traveling from airport to airport and hotel to hotel, I had created a routine. But on this day no part of the routine went well. I got up early to exercise, but the hotel's gym was closed. I went to breakfast for juice and toast, but, this being a Sunday, all they offered was a lavish brunch buffet. The staff had forgotten to deliver the morning news-paper, and the car that was supposed to take me to where I was speak-ing came late, forcing us to rush through traffic and keep the entire audience waiting.

Hunched in the back of the car, I wasn't happy, and I knew why. It wasn't just an interrupted routine; it was failed expectations. I had posted a mental plan about having a good day, and piece by piece the things I expected didn't come true. My desires had been blocked. This happens to everyone. Expectations don't come true, and the result is disappointment. Afterwards I realized that I could have enjoyed my day more if I had approached it without any expectations.

1. I could have been more centered. When you are centered, you aren't so dependent on your circumstances. The ups and downs of everyday events don't throw you off.

2. I didn't need to dictate in advance what a good day would be. One can never see the whole picture. Room needs to be left for the unexpected. In that way, when the unexpected comes, it upsets nothing.

3. I could have let go of outcomes. The only thing any of us can control is our own actions. Outcomes are beyond our control.

4. I could have taken things less personally. Life comes and goes. The universe gives and it takes away.

Nurturing these attitudes in yourself helps you not to build up expectations. I'm not suggesting that you can totally avoid disap-pointment. Our minds are stocked with images of things that we identify with happiness, and by expecting those things, we expose ourselves to letdowns. Yet we also know that a better sort of happiness exists. Next Christmas, which would make you happier, a gift that comes from a list you wrote, or a gift that comes as a complete sur-prise? Your soul doesn't exist to fill a mental list constructed in the past. Its gifts are unexpected. The happiness it brings is fresh because it comes from outside our expectations.

The magic of desire is linked to the freshness of life as it constantly renews itself. The soul isn't a suitor who whispers "I love you" in your ear. The soul has no words, no voice. It expresses love through action, by bestowing the next thing that will give you joy. The next thing may be insignificant; it may be earth-shaking. Only one thing is certain: love awakens the soul and brings its love in return. That's the experience you will have once your boundaries begin to soften. Ultimately, the possibility opens up of a life without any boundaries. It's this possibility we need to explore next.

In Your Life: Letting Your Soul Shine Through

The influence of higher awareness is constant and always beneficial. Like a warm light melting an ice sculpture, it doesn't matter if the ice is carved into a fearsome monster; all that matters is melting it. If you can't feel the warmth of your soul shining through, it's being blocked. Resistance can always be traced back to the mind. These obstacles, being invisible, are difficult to spot. Your mind is expert at hiding from itself, and your ego insists that building boundaries is one of its most important jobs. So the best way to observe what you're doing is through the body. Your body can't fool itself the way your mind can. It has no access to denial. Fear and anger are its responses to the most powerful threats. When your body registers either emotion, some outside force is pushing against your boundaries.

Fear is physically debilitating, and when it turns to terror, it paralyzes. Fear is registered by a tight stomach, cramps, coldness, blood rushing from the head, dizziness, feeling faint, and tightness in the chest. Anger is registered by warmth and flushed skin, tense muscles, a clamped jaw, quick, irregular breathing or loud breathing, a faster heartbeat, and a pounding in the ears.

These are unmistakable signals, but the mind can ignore them anyway. Notice how often a person will say "I'm okay, nothing's wrong" when her body is blatantly contradicting her. You need to trust your body's cues, even when your mind is saying otherwise. Trust begins by recognizing the signature of each emotion. Each one is a sign that you are resisting. An experience is creating stress, and that happens because instead of flowing through you, that experience has hit a barrier. Maybe you can't see what's going on, but your body can feel it. Feeling is the first step of tearing down barriers and no longer needing them.

It's helpful, then, to explore more of these physical cues. When two feelings are related, like anger and hostility or grief and depression, I've given the primary emotion a longer explanation.

Humiliation is like fear in that your body feels weak, but in this case it isn't cold. Your cheeks redden and your skin warms. You shrink and feel smaller. Extreme fear makes you want to run away; humiliation makes you want to disappear. Humiliation lingers in the body and can be triggered by the slightest memory from the past. Someone who has been severely humiliated, especially in childhood, will be listless, unresponsive, and withdrawn; the body will feel chronically weak and helpless.

Embarrassment is mild humiliation. It shows the same physical signs but passes more quickly.

Frustration is like anger, but more bottled up. It feels as if your body wants to be angry but can't find the switch. Movements become rigid, another sign that the outlet is blocked. Frustration can also be anger combined with denial, in which case you will experience signs of denial—averted eyes, quick, dismissive speech, shrugging, tightened jaw muscles, labored breathing. In other words, the person's real feelings are dammed up. Some people show subtle signs of being angry, such as being too restless to sit still. Not all frustration is linked to anger, but even when someone complains of being sexually frustrated, for example, irritability and anger are rarely far away.

Guilt creates a restless feeling, like being trapped and wanting desperately to escape. You feel confined or suffocated; breathing can seem difficult. The chest tightens and wants to explode, to release pent-up guilt as if it were physically trapped. We say that guilt gnaws at you, which the body can register as chronic pressure on the heart.

Shame is another warm feeling, bringing flushed cheeks and warm skin. But there's also a sense of numbness inside that can feel cold and empty. Like humiliation, shame makes you feel smaller; you shrink and want to disappear. Shame is related to guilt, but it feels more like a dead weight, while guilt is a beast that wants to explode out of you.

Anxiety is chronic fear; it's an emotion that weakens the body. The more acute signs of fear may not be present because you've grown used to them; your body has adapted. But the body can't adapt completely, and so the fear creeps out in signs like irritability, tuning out, numbness, and sleeplessness. The body can be listless or restless, which sound like opposites. But when anxiety persists for weeks and months, symptoms have time to shift and adapt to each person's circumstances. In all cases, however, if you lie still and go inward, fear will be present just beneath the surface.

Depression feels cold and heavy, lethargic and lacking in energy. There are many varieties of depression, because like chronic anxiety, this condition can last for weeks, or months, or even years. Your body has time to build up its own unique defenses. For example, someone who is depressed typically feels tired, but that's not always true: high-powered types can continue to function by forcing themselves to be energetic despite their depression. When allied to a sense of hopelessness, depression can make you listless and dull; why move when the situation is hopeless to begin with? Depressed people may complain of being cold all the time. They flounder physically when confronted with challenges, as if confused or helpless. Many people balk when depressed, refusing to react; others lose all motivation. Their bodies signal those attitudes by moving slowly, rigidly, or hesitantly.

Grief is like depression but even more cold and numbing. The body can feel so heavy and listless that the person feels dead while they're still alive.

Hostility is like anger, but needs no trigger to set it off. There are angry cues all the time, combined with a kind of simmering vigilance, alert to the slightest excuse for full-blown rage. The body feels tight, tense, and ready for action.

Arrogance is disguised anger, like hostility, and it is also chronic. One sees signs of it all the time, and the person needs only the slightest trigger to start acting proud, dismissive, and aloof. But arrogance buries its underlying anger deeper than hostility, so deep that this normally warm emotion turns cold. Being bottled up and in control, arrogant people don't explode; instead they deliver a measured dose of cold fury, marked by clenched jaws, a cold stare, and rigid facial expressions.

When you detect these physical cues in your own body, the first step is to trust them. The second is to examine their motivation. Boundaries make you act in ways you aren't fully aware of. Often your ego has an agenda of its own, and it is trying to push that agenda, even though your body isn't buying it. Here are some examples of ego agendas:

Self-importance is an overall strategy for seeming bigger, stronger, more in command or control. The physical giveaways tend to be arrogance and other signs of controlled anger. Signs of frustration indicate that nothing is ever good enough. The body is often rigid, with a stiff neck and head held high; the chest can be stuck out or expanded. Along with these cues, self-important people display typical behaviors of impatience, belligerence, aloofness, and cold dismissal. When challenged, they pontificate; if overmatched, they withdraw and balk.

Prickliness, easily taking offense is the ego's strategy for dealing with fear and insecurity. The person tries to project a self-image that's stronger than he or she actually feels. Therefore, the smallest slight feels like a threat or a wound. There are degrees of this strategy, as with everything the ego does. Curmudgeons are chronically prickly and need no trigger; they feel angry and disgusted all the time. Egotism, which is insecure self-centeredness, always comes with a sense that one is a fraud; therefore, taking offense is the egotist's way of attacking first in order not to be found out.

Criticism and perfectionism constitute another variation on attacking before someone else attacks you. In this case, the critic fears being seen as imperfect. There's an underlying sense of being wrong or defective. The sense of being never good enough is projected outward: "Nothing can be right with you if I'm not right." When our ego adopts this agenda, it thinks it's protecting us from anxiety and humiliation. Perfectionists hold up impossible standards so that nothing can ever be good enough, thereby proving that they are right to feel that they can never be good enough. There's obviously an element of anger here as well, since the critic and perfectionist are attacking their victims, much as they always protest that "it isn't personal." It's always personal—to them.

Dependency is the ego's way of pretending to be helpless because it doesn't want to face its fear. Dependent people cling and act needy. They refuse to take responsibility. They idealize stronger people and try to latch on to them (if only in fantasy, as hero worship). The underlying physical cues are those of anxiety, depression, humiliation. When they are happy, dependent people warm up; they love being loved. When they have no one to lean on, however, they become cold, withdrawn, and depressed. There's often a sense of vagueness about them, because they don't know how to get what they want. They depend on someone else to get it for them, as children do. The body will often show signs of being childlike and immature by being weak, clumsy, uncoordinated, and prone to injury and sickness.

Competitiveness, overachieving, and acting overbearing is a very general ego strategy, one that externalizes fulfillment and makes it dependent on winning. The underlying feeling can be hard to read. It could be anger or fear. It could be anything, really, since the person is so fixated on outer accomplishment that there are no windows looking inward. The physical cues are also hard to read, because competitive people exert constant efforts to be energized, up and running. They are easy to read when they fail, however, since this leads to anger, frustration, and depression. Instead of examining those feelings, the born winner waits them out until he has recharged his batteries and is up again. But no matter how exuberant and energized they appear, overly competitive people secretly know the price they are paying for being number one. Climbing to the top excites them, but they feel exhausted and insecure once they get there, anxious about what tomorrow will bring—which is inevitably newer, younger competitors just like them. In time, winners can wind up baffled and confused. They have built so many inner barriers to protect their "weak" feelings—as they would label them—that when they decide to look inward at last, they have little idea how to go about it.

Failure, underachieving, and checking out is the opposite strategy from being a winner. The ego, never competing or fully engaging, prefers to sit on the sidelines. It lets life pass by while hanging out. The physical cues are generally not hard to spot. Because they are listless, such people show signs of anxiety, a chronic hidden fear that makes them cold, sluggish, limp, undefended, and vulnerable. Their bodies look slumped as if in defeat. The chest is sunken, the posture stooped. Their eyes are averted or look at the ground. There's a general sense that they don't want to be seen or noticed, so their bodies often appear to shrink. It may be that the person is actually holding a job and supporting a family, but inside, their sense of failure is chronic; it makes them feel small, weak, and immature, as if they mysteriously failed to grow up.

To expand in awareness, you must see past these ego agendas and learn to be honest about your motivations. There's a sort of negotiation constantly going on between your ego and your body. When you become aware of what your body is trying to tell you, then your ego can't keep reinforcing its agenda. You have physical proof that you are blocking out the flow of experience, which should be easy, carefree, and spontaneous. So when you see yourself falling back on a fixed ego strategy, see it for what it is, and stop. You must catch yourself at the very moment that you begin to act self-important, dependent, or overbearing. Your ego will kick into its prearranged behavior automatically; like muscles, behaviors have memory. Once you trigger them—even slightly—they jump into action.

Simply by being aware, you can check on your body. There will always be signs of an underlying emotion. Feel that emotion; be with it. Contact allows the physical sensation to dissipate naturally; your

discomfort lessens as your body lets go of distorted or stuck energy
that you have been holding on to. Only in this way can you melt away
your defenses. Unless you are aware, change is impossible. But when
you bring awareness to your body, you can start becoming undefended. Reality starts to be more acceptable as it is, not as you try to
force it to be.

Congratulate yourself for being willing to change. Awareness is
capable of overcoming the most restricted boundaries, because every
boundary is made of nothing but awareness that has decided to contract instead of expand. Also, appreciate your body for its honesty. It
has been letting your soul shine through when your mind refused to.
You are making a connection to your body, and each connection,
however small, brings you closer to your soul as the level of life where
you can reside permanently and with total ease.

Breakthrough #3

Be as Boundless as Your Soul

It takes a major breakthrough to get beyond all boundaries. We are so used to thinking in limited terms that even the soul has become limited. It has become a thing, an object that just happens to be invisible. Look closely at the sentence, "I have a soul." What does "have" mean in that sentence? It seems to mean the same thing as having a house or having a job. It implies ownership, as if your soul belongs to you. If you did possess a soul that way, the following things could also be true:

You could lose your soul.
You could give it away.
You could put a price on it.
You'd know where your soul is located.
You could compare yours with someone else's.

These are just a few of the troubling implications that stem from thinking that the soul is an invisible object. You can find someone to believe in every item on the list. Most cultures have legends about losing one's soul, selling it to the devil, or having demons run away with it. Even today, losing your soul stands as a very real threat to devout Christians. We need to find an alternative idea, because as soon as souls can be lost or saved, blessed or condemned, they become objects. The time has come to make a breakthrough and treat the soul as it really is.

In place of a soul that you *own*, which is mythical, there's an unbounded soul that exists everywhere. The soul is primarily a link to the infinite. It consists of pure awareness, the raw stuff from which all your thoughts, sensations, wishes, dreams, and visions are made. Think of white, the purest hue. White doesn't look to the eye as if all colors could be derived from it. You would suppose the opposite, that no colors could be extracted, since white itself has no color. Pure awareness goes even further. It isn't a thought, yet all thoughts come from it. It isn't a sensation, yet the senses derive from it. In fact, pure awareness lies beyond any experience in space and time. It has no beginning or end. Nothing can bind or enclose it, any more than you could enclose all the energy that erupted in the Big Bang. Yet the influence of the soul permeates all of creation. The unbounded soul flows in, around, and through you. Indeed, it is the real you because it's your source.

I think religions fell back on personalizing the soul as "mine" or "yours" because just as an infinite God boggles the mind, so does the unbounded soul. Something more manageable was needed. Hence a personal God who sits above the clouds and looks down on his children, to whom he has provided a personal soul that fits neatly inside the heart. Reducing the soul to a piece of private property makes it easier to handle, but it distorts reality. Let's try to reclaim reality. Can you and I be as unbounded as our souls? I think we can. That's exactly where our journey is taking us. If living inside boundaries creates limitation and suffering, the only alternative is living outside them. There lies freedom from suffering; there lies true fulfillment. The unbounded soul can't be lost or saved, it can't be denied or evicted by God, because God is made of the same pure awareness.

When you give up the idea of "my soul," you can participate in an unbounded creation. Countless people don't realize that such a choice exists; many more wouldn't choose an unbounded life if it was offered. Living within boundaries offers a sense of security. But this turns out to be an either/or choice. Let me illustrate.

There's a clever tactic reportedly used by the indigenous Bushmen of South Africa to find water. In the desert regions that the Bushmen have long inhabited—they are thought to be the oldest strain of humanity still existing—water is scarce and difficult to find in the dry season. But one creature that can always locate the most hidden springs and pools is the baboon. The Bushmen trick baboons into showing them where the water is by placing some choice nuts inside a hollow tree. The opening to this cache is barely large enough for the baboon to stick its paw in. When it reaches for the nuts and grabs a handful, the animal can't get its closed first back out again. The baboon is too greedy to let go of the nuts, and so it is trapped. Hours go by, and eventually the baboon is too thirsty to stay. It lets go of the nuts and immediately runs to find water, with the lurking Bushmen following. The baboon has become their unwitting guide.

There's a moral here about the soul. As long as the baboon holds on to what it wants, it's trapped. But as soon as it lets go, it wins its freedom. So long as you cling to anything by saying "mine," you can't be free. Your soul isn't a thing you can cling to and make your own. Caught in the Bushmen's trap, you can only win your freedom by letting go. The mystery of the unbounded soul is wrapped up in those two issues: how much you want to be free, and how to let go.

How do you let go?

As a practical matter, people are torn between holding on and letting go. In our society, holding on is seen in a positive light: we hold on to our dreams, our hopes, our livelihood, our faith. But there's a suspicious trace of ego here. The ego holds on too long and for the wrong reasons. It has a vested interest in being right. Is it right to live behind boundaries? You will never know until you challenge your ego's certainty. That's why letting go is rarely simple: consider how many miserable relationships persist because one spouse or the other insists on proving that he or she is right Pain and suffering aren't strong enough to trump the desire to be right. The endless arguments among the world's faiths, which regularly erupt in crusades, jihads, and other forms of religious violence, attest to this. All religions preach peace, and so warring over peace destroys the very value being defended. Every religion believes that divine love should be followed as a model on earth, but love evaporates in the midst of conflict.

Yet living from the level of the soul is impossible without letting
go. This is a choice you make eventually. In daily life, this either/or
choice is well defined. Here's what the two sides look like.

SOUL	EGO
Accepting	*Rejecting*
Approving	*Critical*
Cooperating	*Opposing*
Detached	*Clinging*
Calm	*Agitated*
Forgiving	*Resentful*
Selfless	*Selfish*
Peaceful	*Conflicted*
Nonjudgmental	*Judgmental*

Your soul is just as much a part of you as your ego. Given a
simple choice, all of us would choose the soul's way. We would rather
accept than reject; we'd want to be peaceful rather than agitated. But
life brings difficulties, and to cope with those difficulties we are forced
to make choices that aren't simple. What if your house was robbed
and the police caught a couple of teenagers with the flat-screen television they stole? You have your property back. Would you choose not
to prosecute? What if they caught the teenagers, but your television
had already been fenced? Would you be more inclined to prosecute?
These negotiations between mercy and punishment are symbolic of
the fork in the road that presents itself whenever the ego would go
one way and the soul the other.

The most common everyday actions move you away from your
soul. Today or tomorrow you might

reject an experience in advance
criticize someone else or yourself
oppose a new idea
cling to your point of view

feel *agitated* inside

resent the position you've been put in

raise the level of *conflict* in the situation

consider your own *selfish* interests before anything else

cast *judgment* and blame on others

In each situation the ego is being reinforced. Of course, everyone falls back upon these responses without thinking. Or if they think, they feel justified in choosing the ego. But the fixed, stubborn attitude that results is very damaging. All of us have been maddened by people who take their egos to extremes, who are as predictable as clocks because no matter what you say or do, they never alter in their opposition, stubbornness, and selfishness. Yet the same tendencies are preventing you from letting go, too.

It's not that your ego has a totally negative agenda. Under normal circumstances it doesn't. Mainly it acts out of self-protection. Some people—a rare few—have consciously learned how to cope with the world without protecting themselves. They rely on a higher power to protect them, and that's what you and I must learn to do. Otherwise we'll never get outside our defenses. We aren't called upon to be saintly. It's not about whether you are a good person or not. It just needs to sink in that letting go is the path to everything.

Let's see why letting go is so difficult. Think back to the last occasion when you rejected somebody because he or she disagreed with you. Or feel inside what it's like to refuse your cooperation because you have a powerful urge to oppose. Everyday existence brings up these urges in hundreds of small and large ways. Your ego keeps reinforcing the same argument over and over: *Look out for number one. Nobody else is going to stand up for you. You can't afford to sacrifice what you want.*

Psychologically, these reactions aren't about the present but the past. Your ego is urging you to think and act like a damaged child. Such a child only wants what it wants. It has no ability to see beyond the immediate moment, and when it doesn't get what it wants, a damaged child pouts, balks, and throws tantrums. I know that the phrase "inner child" has been romanticized as an ideal of innocence and love. That child, too, exists in all of us; you will see it anytime that the soul shines through. But your inner child has a shadow self that embodies the tactics of an angry, wounded, selfish infant. When your ego dips into those shadow energies, they impel you to act in very regressive ways.

It's hard, as a well-adjusted adult, to face the fact that you are harboring a shadow that's not only destructive but childish and irrational, too. Yet something positive is close at hand once you make it through the shadows. Every spiritual tradition invokes our so-called higher self, the side of human nature that the soul stands for. We recognize ourselves in the love Jesus preached, and in the compassion espoused by Buddha. Every spiritual tradition also makes it clear that our so-called lower nature, identified with sin and ignorance, must be transformed. Unfortunately, the choice is presented in a way that's unhelpful. How can you adopt love when you are told at the same time that your lower nature is sinful? Condemning the lower self is the opposite of love. How can you adopt peace when you are told at the same time to fight against temptation? You wind up being trapped in your divided nature instead of healing it.

As a practical matter, the part of yourself that you judge against isn't going to change. It has no motivation to cooperate—quite the opposite, in fact. Whatever you fight against digs in even more deeply. After all, you are threatening its survival. Let me offer an example from politics, since the outer world is easier for most of us to understand than the inner self. In the United States, deep divisiveness developed between people who supported the second war in Iraq and those who opposed it. Eventually the arguments against the war became convincing, if not overwhelming. As an experiment, a group of pro-war voters were put in a room and asked to rate their support on a scale from 1 to 10. They were then given a talk on the reasons for being against the war. The year was 2008, five years into the Iraqi conflict, so there was a mountain of objective reporting about the most contentious issues, such as weapons of mass destruction, the threat of terrorism, civilian casualties, and so on.

The experimenters presented the antiwar position as factually as possible, being deliberately dispassionate. At the end of the lecture the group was asked to rate their pro-war position a second time on a scale of 1 to 10. The results might startle you, but the group actually became more pro-war. The reason wasn't that they necessarily disbelieved the antiwar facts. They just didn't like having their noses rubbed in their mistakes.

Likewise, the parts of yourself that feel judged against will not relent. They will try to persuade you even harder to be selfish, judgmental, and resentful whenever you face outside opposition. Spiritual traditions haven't taken into account that there's a process involved in weaning the ego from its self-defeating ways. By putting the issue in terms of morality, sin, and the threat of God's wrath, Christianity has taken the opposite of an effective approach. Buddhism is less inclined to be moralistic, and it possesses an extremely subtle system of psychology. But when simplified, the practice of Buddhism gets reduced to "ego death," a direct assault upon the ego as the source of ignorance and illusion.

The whole business of making a stark contrast between the lower and higher self is futile to begin with. There is no separate, all-good, all-wise part of you that you must either win or lose. Life is one flow of awareness. No aspect of you was constructed out of anything else. Fear and anger are actually made from the same pure awareness as love and compassion; erecting a barrier between ego and soul fails to recognize this simple fact. In the end, letting go is achieved not by condemning what's bad in yourself and throwing it away, but by a process that brings opposites together. Your ego must see that it belongs to the same reality as your soul. It needs to find so much in common with your soul that it lets go of its selfish agenda in favor of a better way of life.

Jordan's story

Letting go is often a last resort, but then something magical can happen. Invisible powers that you never expected can come to your aid.

Jordan is a successful career woman in her late thirties, and she has just saved a marriage she had almost given up on. "Mike wasn't my soul mate. We didn't fall in love at first sight," Jordan said. "We met at work, and he asked me out several times before I said yes. I had to learn to love him, but once I did, it felt very real.

"A year later we took the plunge. Mike was twenty-nine, I was twenty-six. We were in love, but we also sat down and discussed what we wanted out of this marriage. So when all the trouble began, it really caught me off guard."

"How did it begin?" I asked.

"I couldn't tell you exactly," Jordan said. "But Mike started behaving like my father, a man who never listens and never gives in. I had married Mike because he seemed to be the exact opposite. Mike was gentle and open. He listened. But then he changed. We started fighting a lot, and I got very upset."

"Did he accuse *you* of changing?" I asked.

"He got very bitter about it. I never gave him enough space, he said. But 'space' doesn't mean brooding about your work for hours on end and pushing me away when I wanted to make up after a fight. Mike would hold me for a minute, maybe two. But I could tell he wanted to be alone, to go back to his computer or his video games."

"So what did you do?" I asked.

"I didn't sink into despair. I told Mike that if we loved each other, we should be able to ask for what we wanted emotionally. I'm not needy, but for God's sake, if I felt like crying or wanting to be held, he barely responded."

"Maybe he saw your emotions as weak, or as a threat," I suggested.

Jordan agreed. "Mike's scared of emotions, and he can't stand weakness. I was expected to make him feel like a winner. Anything else was a betrayal. I should have seen that sooner. Mike came from a very rigid family where nobody thought that showing your feelings was a positive thing."

"Eventually you considered leaving him?" I asked.

"It happened one evening. He was eating dinner in front of the football game, and no matter what I said, he barely nodded. I stood up and told him to turn off the damn TV. He just gave this little dismissive laugh. I thought to myself, 'I'm not turning into a cliché. I've got my whole life to live.'

"It took me a long time to stop feeling sorry for myself. But I had been reading a lot about self-development, and one thing I'd read stuck with me: Accept total responsibility for your own life."

"What did that mean to you?" I asked.

"What it didn't mean," said Jordan, shaking her head, "is that everything was my fault. I was encouraged to looked at things more positively. I was the creator of my own life. If I wanted my life to change, the means were inside of me. Once I stopped pitying myself, I realized that this was a test. Mike was in total denial. Could I save the marriage myself? Think what a triumph that would be. I didn't consult Mike or anybody else. This was my own secret project. So I started in on it."

"What did you do?"

"I had learned a new term, 'reactive mind'; this is the mode you're in when you constantly react to the other person, which gives them power over you. When Mike pushed my buttons, arguing over who was right and who was wrong, I couldn't help but react. When I was growing up, my mother only had two ways of dealing with a bad situation. She either tried to fix it or she put up with it. There's a third way, which is to leave until you're able to cope. So instead of getting angry at Mike or sulking or complaining, I kept my cool, and as soon as I could, I'd get away and be with myself."

"What did you do then?"

"I processed my feelings on my own. The reactive mind is quick to respond, but when your first reaction dies down, other responses have room to show up. I examined anger as my issue, not Mike's fault; self-pity came from me, not from what Mike did to me. When Mike and I fought, everything was about defending myself, because he can't stand to lose. The great thing about learning that you can look inside yourself is that you can give up being so defensive."

"How did your husband react?" I asked.

"At first Mike didn't like that I was holding back. He thought that by not fighting back I was acting superior. But that didn't last long. After I dealt with my feelings, I went back in to be with him, and he liked the fact that I didn't return with resentment or bottled-up frustration."

"Once you quit tugging at your end of the rope," I said, "there was no more tug-of-war."

"That was a tough lesson to learn, but yes. Also, we hate in others what we deny in ourselves. I hated it when Mike would come home and instantly start complaining that he wanted a warm meal and a loving wife, two things I wasn't providing. I felt attacked. But then I asked myself if I wasn't passively attacking him by withholding those things. I was defying him, which made my ego feel good, but all it led to was a hostile standoff."

"You don't mean that giving in to Mike was the solution, do you?" I said.

"In a way, yes, that's what I do mean," said Jordan. "I surrendered. I gave of myself. But what made that a positive thing was that first I got to the place inside myself where surrender wasn't failure. Surrender can mean that you lost the battle. But it can also mean that you are surrendering to love instead of hate." She laughed. "All right, I gritted my teeth the first couple of times that I met Mike at the door with a kiss and the smell of fresh-baked bread in the background. But honestly, before long I felt very good about myself."

Jordan's rescue mission for her marriage unfolded in many other ways, but we had covered the critical part, learning how to let go. This is more than a relationship strategy; a deep personal shift is involved. You release yourself from ego-bound reactions—what some call the reactive mind—and allow events to unfold without a preset program. The risks can be terrifying. Everyone has a voice inside warning that to surrender is a sign of weakness. Jordan had downplayed the fear that arises in such situations. I asked her if things had been at all frightening for her.

"That's what makes it so wonderful to come out the other side," she said. "No one knows the terror you go through. Being strong enough to risk your sense of pride, your image of yourself as a woman who won't be trampled on—only somebody who's gone through it knows how difficult that is."

I agreed. The negative connotations of surrender have been drummed into us. We equate it not only with losing the battle, but with weakness and lack of self-respect. In this particular case, surrender of the feminine to the masculine raises every imaginable red flag.

"Were you conscious of that?" I asked Jordan.

"Oh yes. I had lots of fights with myself, lots of self-doubt. But the bottom line was that I wasn't surrendering to Mike. I was surrendering to the truth, and the truth is that I want to love and be loved. I was taking responsibility for my truth, which brings incredible personal power if you can do it."

Jordan feels proud that she got past all her inner resistance, and her pride is justified. Her marriage is intact and has blossomed into a far more secure love than she knew before. The part that no one else knows, the real mystery, is that when she changed, everything changed. Her husband stopped doing all the things she resented. He looked at her with different eyes, as if he was rediscovering the woman he fell in love with.

Jordan didn't have to ask him to do that; it just happened. How? To begin with, there's a deep connection when two people love each other. We know instinctively whether that connection is working or is broken. The connection must be restored at a deep level, a place the ego can't reach. Here the element of the soul is inescapable. But why should another person, or an entire situation, change just because you do? If each of us owned a soul like private property, then change would happen one person at a time. But the unbounded soul connects everyone. Its influence is felt everywhere. So, when you change your behavior at the level of the soul, the whole dance must change along with you.

In Your Life: "You're Not Me"

Life brings many situations where letting go isn't easy. Fortunately, there's one strategy that always works. Instead of focusing on your reaction in the moment, step back and reassert who you really are. The real you has no agenda. It lives in the present; it responds to life openly. Therefore the attitude you need to take to any pre-programmed response—which is all your ego has to offer—is always the same: "You're not me." Let fear, anger, jealousy, resentment, victimization, or any conditioned reaction arise. Don't oppose it. Yet the minute you become aware of it, say, "You're not me."

With one stroke you accomplish two things. You put the ego on notice that you've seen through its game, and you call upon your real self to help you. If your soul is the real you, then it possesses the power to transform you, once you open yourself to it. You will know that you are responding from the soul level whenever you do the following:

Accept the experience that's in front of you.
Approve of other people and yourself.
Cooperate with the solution at hand.
Detach yourself from negative influences.
Remain *calm* in the face of stress.
Forgive those who offend or wrong you.
Approach the situation *selflessly*, with fairness to all.
Exert a *peaceful* influence.
Take a *nonjudgmental* attitude, making no one else feel wrong.

These responses can't be forced or planned ahead—not if you genuinely want to be transformed. It's self-defeating to adopt them simply because you think they make you look good. Maddening as it is to run into people who are stubbornly petty and selfish, forced virtue can be just as maddening. The problem is that what is really needed—letting go—hasn't happened. The publicly virtuous have simply found a new ego agenda that makes them look better than they are.

When you find yourself reacting from ego, stop and say, "You're not me." Then what? There are four steps that allow your soul to bring in a new response.

1. Remain centered.
2. Be clear.
3. Expect the best.
4. Watch and wait.

1. Remain centered. By now most people know the value of being centered; it's a state of calm and stability. When you aren't centered, you feel scattered and off-kilter. Feelings fight against each other. There's no stability in your reactions because the next event can pull you this way or that. Panic is the ultimate state of not being centered, but there are many milder ones, such as distraction, restlessness, confusion, anxiety, and disorientation. Unfortunately, knowing that it's better to be centered isn't the same as getting there.

Where is this center? For some it's the middle of the chest, or the heart itself. For others it's the solar plexus, or simply a general sense of "going inside." I'd suggest, however, that the center isn't physical. Your heart can't be your center when it's racing or in pain. Your solar plexus can't be your center when your intestines are in a knot. The body always reflects consciousness, therefore your center is in awareness. This points us in the right direction, but awareness is always shifting, so the question is, where can you find calmness and peace that cannot be shaken?

You won't be surprised, I'm sure, to hear that absolute calm and peace are located at the soul level, which is reached through meditation. We have discussed this, but it bears repeating that no matter who you are or in whatever crisis, this place of peace and calm is never shattered. Even to come near is to experience its effects. When you want to seek your center, find a quiet place where you cannot be disturbed. Close your eyes and feel the part of your body that feels stressed. Breathing easily and regularly, release the disturbed energy from that part of the body.

Quite often your mind will contain stressed thoughts. These will usually disappear once you settle your body down. If they don't, then breathe out the energy that lies behind those thoughts, meaning the energy of fear and anxiety. There's more than one way to do that.

Through the crown chakra*:* In yoga, the top of the head is considered an energy center, or *chakra*. It's an effective place for releasing energy. Close your eyes and see a beam of white light extending up through your head and exiting through a tiny opening in the crown. The beam of light is narrow, but it gathers all the swirling thoughts in your head and projects them out in one stream through the crown chakra—you might visualize your thoughts as swirling smoke that the beam of light gathers up and transports away.

Breathing: Blow out in a a steady exhale—like blowing out a birthday candle, but slower. Watch the white light of your exhalation streaming upward, taking all your stressed thoughts with it. Watch the light going up and up beyond the room until you can't see it anymore.

Toning: It also helps to make a high tone at the same time as you breathe out, a soft "Eeeee" sound. The first time or two, you may find this exercise strange, but even if you can't manage the toning or breathing the first time you try, just using the beam of white light to carry energy up and out of the body can be effective on its own.

2. Be clear. It takes mental clarity to let go. You must be able to tell the true from the false, so you can identify what you want to let go. When you are afraid, fear seems to *be* you. When you are angry, anger takes you over. But behind this drama and emotional turmoil, the real you is right there, waiting for you to connect to yourself.

I can illustrate this best through the story of Jacob, a man who came to see me after suffering from depression his entire adult life; he's now fifty. Jacob wasn't asking for therapy. He wanted a handle on how to achieve real change. I told him that depression can be overcome by letting it go. To do that, he had to clarify a few basic things.

"Let's see how you feel about your depression," I began. "Imagine that it has taken the shape of a person who walks in the door and sits down on a chair facing you."

Jacob closed his eyes and started to visualize. After a few minutes he told me that he saw his depression as a gnarled, hunched-over old man who had shuffled into the room. The old man was smelly and dressed in filthy army fatigues.

"Good," I said. 'Now that you see him, how do you feel about him?" Jacob said he felt bad. "Don't tell me," I said. "Tell him."

At first Jacob was hesitant. But with a bit of coaxing, he told the old man, "You scare me to death, and you exhaust me. My mind races with anxiety, and while others see me as someone listless and passive, I feel like I'm wrestling with a demon every moment of the day." Once he got started, Jacob's accusations intensified. He poured out his feelings of hostility and anguish. He spoke bitterly of how impossible it was for him to express his pain, so helpless did the gnarled old man make him feel.

I let Jacob get everything out, until he was spent. 'You will never get past your depression unless you let this old man inside you go," I said. "To the extent that you push this old man away and revile him, he will remain the same. The problem has been turned into a part of yourself, but it's not who you really are."

Jacob grew quiet. We were old friends, so I could talk to him intimately. I told him that he didn't think he was holding on to his depression, but this old man was an aspect of himself. It was a creation of a distorted self-image, and over the years it had gained so much energy that it seemed to have a life of its own.

"Your depression makes you feel helpless because you believe that you have no choice. You can't remember not being depressed. In reality, you do have a choice. You can negotiate with the old man and tell him that it's time to leave. You can release the energy of depression. You can meditate and find the level inside your awareness that isn't depressed. But if you continue to think that being depressed is a permanent part of you, that's a choice, too. You need to take responsibility for it." I was trying to give Jacob enough clarity to face his depression, to say to it, "You're not me."

This talk was only the beginning. Off and on we made contact again, then Jacob dropped out of sight for a while. Recently he resurfaced, and it was obvious that he was no longer depressed. His energy was stronger and more positive. "Did that one conversation turn the tide?" I asked him.

"I think so," Jacob said with quiet conviction. "The timing must have been just right, because I surrendered. The fight went out of me. I had been leading myself on with the hope that one day I'd defeat my depression. But you were right. Hating my depression had done absolutely no good."

During the time that I hadn't seen him, Jacob had pulled his life together. He entered into a serious relationship; he began to work for a spiritual cause he believed in. He decided to ignore his depression and minimize the hold it had over him. But the critical thing was a change of attitude. He began to accept himself, to see that depression wasn't his real self.

"I got clear about a lot of things. I became gentler and easier with myself. I stopped pushing and judging myself. It took time. Nothing happened all at once. But as I opened up a space inside myself, something new entered the picture. I gave my mind permission to settle down, and it quit racing so much. It quit being so desperate. Once I felt calmer, it was like slowly waking up. The world got brighter. Gradually, being happy became possible. That's the best way that I can put it."

Clarity, because it's internal, brings home the truth that can't be absorbed when you are confused or agitated. You see that you can't change what you hate in yourself. Many people who suffer have firsthand experience with the futility of warring with themselves. The breakthrough comes when they accept that the thing they hate has no real independent existence. *This is not me. It's how I am temporarily. It's my energy until I let it go.*

If you are an alcoholic and say, "Drinking is who I am. Put up with it," you aren't moving toward healing. Your defensiveness is a secret form of helplessness. Deep down, you think change is doomed to fail. What's needed is a different attitude, or rather no attitude. You become clear that there's a bundle of energy, emotions, habits, and feelings to let go of, and that's all. Naturally, one moment of clarity doesn't shift everything. What took years to develop takes time to undo. But with clarity comes acceptance, and even a small step toward acceptance opens a channel to the soul.

3. Expect the best. You don't let go so that something good might happen. You let go so that the very best in yourself, your soul, can merge with you. By itself, letting go of a bit of anger, a bit of fear, a bit of resentment, might seem tiny. I'd reframe the situation. Imagine that you are used to living in a small, cramped house. You've become so used to this claustrophobic space that you almost never go outside. Yet there are carefree moments when you think it would be nice to experience a wider world. So you open the door, and as you step outside, you confront a vast landscape, filled with light and extending to infinity in all directions.

Ah, you think, here is joy and love. Here is real fulfillment. So you roam outside, wanting to abide in this land of light forever. Yet after a while you get tired of all this love and joy. Somehow the space outside is too vast, the horizon too infinite. You miss your familiar house, and it pulls you back. So you return, and it feels safe to be back. You resume your familiar existence. For a time you're content again, but you keep remembering that vast, unlimited space outside. Once again you step out, and this time you stay there longer. Your sense of love and joy isn't so tiring. The space outside is still infinite, but that doesn't frighten you so much. The light that shines everywhere isn't so blinding, and you resolve that this time you will abide here forever.

This is a parable about the ego and the soul. The ego is your safe house; the soul is the unbounded space outside. Every time you feel even a moment of joy and love, freedom and bliss, you have stepped into the land of light. You feel so wonderful that you want to keep the experience going, the way two infatuated lovers never want to be apart. But your ego, your safe house, calls you back. This pattern of coming and going is how letting go works. It takes repeated exposure to the unbounded soul for you to know that it is real. But your old conditioning will keep pulling you back. In time, your trips outside will last longer and feel more comfortable. Your soul is starting to seep into you; with this merging you begin to understand that you can live in the unbounded permanently. It becomes more natural than your safe house because in the unbounded you are the real you.

Therefore, expecting the best isn't about wishful thinking or optimism. It's about recognizing in advance that your goal is attainable. The unbounded soul is experienced, however faintly, in every impulse of the soul. This counters the prevailing attitude in psychology that happiness is a temporary state stumbled upon by accident. I find that attitude deplorable. To declare that love and joy, the primal components of happiness, are occasional is a teaching born of desperation. Keep in mind the image of the safe house and the land of light that surrounds it. No one will ever force you to let go of the limited space you occupy, but you always have the choice to seek the infinite, because that is who you are.

4. Watch and wait. Surrendering in battle happens once, at the very end. Surrendering on the spiritual path happens over and over, and it never ends. For this reason, watching and waiting isn't a passive act. It's not an exercise in patience, or a kind of down time until the big event starts. The moment you let go of some old habit or conditioning, the instant you catch yourself in a programmed reaction, the self shifts. As casually as we use the word *self,* it isn't a simple thing but a complex, dynamic system. Your self is a micro universe mirroring the macro universe. Countless forces are moving through it. As fluid as air, the self changes with every shift in awareness.

Therefore, whenever you let go, you are subtracting something old from the universe and adding something new. The old is dark energy and distorted patterns from the past. These are dead bits that got stuck inside the self's system. Having no way to eject them, you worked around them. You adjusted to negative elements in yourself—usually through denial and by pushing these elements down out of sight—because you assumed that you had to. Letting go isn't an option until you learn how to make it an option. Once you do let them go, the negative energies depart permanently.

Which allows something new to enter. What will it be? That's what watching and waiting reveals. Think of what happens when you breathe in. New oxygen atoms enter your bloodstream, but where they go isn't predetermined. An oxygen atom can wind up in any one of billions of cells. Its destination is determined by which cell needs it the most. The same is true of you. When you open space for the soul by letting go of old energies, the part of you in greatest need, the part that wants most eagerly to grow or most seriously wants healing, will benefit.

To take an example on a larger scale, I've often thought that Jesus became the greatest teacher of love because that's what his audience needed most. They weren't starved for divine wisdom, spiritual discipline, or enlightenment—all of which became dominant in other traditions like Buddhism. At a more human level, Jesus' listeners wanted God's love, and so that's what they absorbed. No doubt Jesus was as complete a teacher as Buddha. He taught the way to higher consciousness, even enlightenment. But that part has to be searched out in the corners of his teaching; the foreground is occupied by love in every form.

To know what your soul is, you must follow the path it takes as it enters you. Will it make you more loving and kind? Will it make you more devout and worshipful? Any quality can be imparted by the soul—strength, truth, beauty, or faith. But these aren't laid on like a coat of paint. Rather, they enter you as oxygen enters your body, seeking out what is most needed. We speak of being filled with spirit, as if all it takes is pumping a person up the way you pump up a bicycle tire. In reality, spirit is awareness traveling to places where awareness is lacking. It speeds your growth enormously if you are there to receive the healing when it arrives.

Too often, people don't watch and wait. They miss what's really happening inside them. They fixate on wishes and fantasies, and while their attention is distracted, the real thing passes them by. I love the story of Harold Arlen, a famous Hollywood composer in the golden era of movies, who was assigned to write the music for *The Wizard of Oz*. Arlen worked steadily at it, and he thought he had done a good job. But one song was lacking, the special one that he knew the score needed, the topper. Nothing would come, so Arlen gave up for the day and took his wife to lunch. On the way down Sunset Boulevard he suddenly told his wife, who was at the wheel, to pull over. Arlen scribbled some notes on a scrap of paper, which turned out to be the music for a song called "Somewhere Over the Rainbow."

In many ways, artists and creators know best how to receive the soul, because they attune themselves to inspiration. Inspiration doesn't happen randomly. It's always a matter of call and response. The need goes out, and the solution appears. So take a creative attitude toward your own inner growth. Be aware of your need and watch for the response. When asked how he came up with such great music, Harold Arlen said, "I drift, wait, and obey." It wouldn't hurt to take heed of that credo, which is simple but profound.

Breakthrough #4

The Fruit of Surrender Is Grace

A breakthrough can lead you to the ultimate surrender. Because letting go is a process, it eventually comes to an end. But this end point is very different from anything one would anticipate. You won't be the person you see in the mirror today. That person goes through life with endless needs. In the ultimate surrender, you give up all needs. For the first time you will be able to say, "I am enough." You will find yourself in a world where everything fits together as it should.

A completely new self can't be imagined in advance. A young child has no idea that the future will bring the drastic changes triggered by puberty. It would be confusing to try to understand that until the experience is at hand (there's confusion enough when that moment arrives). Letting go of childhood comes naturally, if you are lucky. Letting go of your adult identity is much more difficult. We have no maps to guide us, although there is certainly a call from the world's great spiritual teachers. Saint Paul compares it to growing up. "When I was a child, I spoke like a child, I thought like a child, I reasoned like a child; when I became an adult, I put an end to childish ways."

Going from child to adult means changing your identity, but Paul is pointing to a far more shattering kind of transformation. He says, "Pursue love and strive for the spiritual gifts," and then holds out a vision of what will happen if someone heeds the call.

Love is patient; love is kind; love is not envious or boastful or arrogant or rude. It does not insist on its own way; it is not irritable or resentful; it does not rejoice in wrongdoing, but rejoices in the truth. It bears all things, believes all things, hopes all things, endures all things. (I CORINTHIANS 13: 4–7)

Paul was well aware that he was calling for supernatural change. All of human nature would be transformed, and the only power capable of doing that was grace. You cannot find the word "grace" in the Bible without its connotations close by—abundance, purity, unconditional love, a gift freely given. There's something universal here that goes beyond Judeo-Christianity. By letting go completely, a person can achieve a new identity. The fruit of surrender is grace, the all-embracing power of God.

Grace is the invisible influence of the divine. Once it enters a person's life, the old tools that we have used to run our lives—reason, logic, effort, planning, forethought, discipline—are discarded like the training wheels of a bicycle. But the actual process is shadowy and amorphous. Grace is associated with mercy and forgiveness, but in reality, if you strip it of religious overtones, grace is unbounded awareness.

Grace abolishes life's limitations. There is nothing to fear, nothing to be guilty of. The whole issue of good versus evil disappears. Peace is no longer a dream to be chased, but an innate quality of the heart. These things are the result not of supernatural intervention, but of coming to the end of a process. The word *grace* occurs almost a hundred times in the Old Testament, but, curiously, Jesus doesn't use it even once. One explanation is that we meet Jesus after he has come to the end of the process of finding his unbounded self; he is unique that way.

Grace, like the soul itself, steps down God's infinite power to human scale. It carries more than a whiff of magic, as befits a total transformation. The human mind barely grasps how a caterpillar can transform into a butterfly, much less the miracle of how human beings are transformed by grace. Somehow nothing more is required except surrender. But the process of being born again is recorded in every culture, so let's see if we can come closer to understanding it.

Self-transformation

Before it is touched by grace, human nature is fallen, corrupt, sinful, impure, ignorant, guilty, and blind—those are the traditional terms in Judeo-Christianity. What makes them unhelpful is that they are based on morality. The word *boundary* is neutral; it simply refers to a state of limitation. If you take a person and force him to live in severe limitation—say, in a dungeon—all kinds of problems will develop, from paranoia to delusion. But they aren't because the prisoner is morally defective. They result from being bound up. The difference between a prisoner captive in his cell and you or me is that we have voluntarily chosen to live inside our boundaries. The part of our selves that made this choice is the ego.

The ego is your familiar self, the "I" that goes through the world and deals with everyday events. As long as this self feels satisfied, there's no overriding reason to seek the soul. But is life satisfying? Every great spiritual teacher begins with the assumption that it isn't. Jesus and Buddha confronted a world where ordinary people were beset by disease and poverty. Simply to survive being born and then live to age thirty was a major challenge. It wasn't difficult to convince such an audience that everyday life was steeped in suffering. That problem remains constant, even in modern societies that have made substantial inroads against disease, poverty, and hunger.

Buddha and Jesus weren't concerned with the material causes of suffering. Instead, they traced the cause to its very root, the "I" that handles everyday life. That "I" is a false identity, they said. It masks the real self, which can only be found at the soul level. But this diagnosis didn't lead to anything like a quick cure. The self isn't like a car that can be taken apart and rebuilt as a better model. "I" has an agenda. It thinks it knows how to run everyday life, and when threatened with disassembly, it fights back—after all, survival itself is at stake. For this reason, ego became the great enemy of change (more in the East than the West; in the West, sin and evil took on that role, again for moral reasons). It became obvious that the ego was a subtle opponent, because it had become so pervasive. A person's identity isn't like a cloak that can be taken off. Transforming your identity is more like performing surgery on yourself; you must act as both doctor and patient. This is an impossible task in the physical world, but entirely possible in awareness.

Awareness looks at itself, and when it does, it can search out flaws and fix them. The reason it can mend itself is that only awareness is involved. There is no need to go outside the self, no need to be asleep to block the pain, and no need for violence against the body.

Before surgery begins, you need a disease or defect. The ego, for all its claims to running everyday life, has a glaring defect. Its vision of life is unworkable. What it promises as a completely fulfilling life is an illusion, a will-o'-the-wisp you can chase all your life without ever laying hands on it. When you become aware of this defect, the result is fatal for the ego. It can't compete with the soul's vision of fulfillment. We have all been conditioned to believe that it's the ego that is practical and realistic in its approach to life, while the soul is unattainable and detached from everyday affairs. But that is a complete reversal of the truth. Let me illustrate.

Two Visions of Fulfillment

The ego's vision:

I have everything I need to be comfortable.
I am serene because bad things can't come near me.
Through hard work, anything can be achieved.
I measure myself by my accomplishments.
I win much more often than I lose.
I have a strong self-image.
Because I'm attractive, I win the attention of the opposite sex.
When I find the perfect love, it will be on my terms.

The soul's vision:

I am everything I need.
I am secure because I have nothing to fear in myself.
The flow of life's abundance brings me everything.
I do not measure myself by any external standard.

Giving is more important than winning.

I have no self-image; I am beyond images.

Other people are attracted to me as soul to soul.

I can find perfect love, because I have discovered it first in myself.

It's fair to say, I think, that the second vision describes life in a state of grace. It stands for life transformed, not life as presided over by the ego. Yet, looking at the two choices, most people would find the ego's version more reasonable. For one thing, they are already quite used to it. Familiarity, added to inertia, keeps most of us doing the same things every day. But that aside, what makes the ego's path to fulfillment seem easy is that it is based on improving the conditions of life step by step. If you have a modest job today, it will become more important tomorrow. A small first home will one day turn into a larger home. If you run into problems or obstacles along the way, they can be overcome. Hard work, diligence, loyalty, and faith in progress combine to make life better.

This is the ego's version of personal growth: however limited your life may be, in time it will steadily get better. Yet this vision, so focused on externals, ignores what's actually happening with the inner person. There is no correlation between fulfillment and external progress. A country as impoverished as Nigeria ranks higher among societies on a scale of happiness than the United States (as measured by polls that ask people how happy they are). As far as money goes, people get happier as they rise above the level of poverty, but once the basic wants of life are secure, adding more money actually *decreases* one's chance of being happy. Studies of people who have won the lottery find that within a year or two, not only are they worse off materially, but the majority say they wish they had never won in the first place. (Needless to say, these findings are not widely promoted by the lotteries themselves.)

We pay dearly for latching on to externals as the measure of who we are. Downturns in the economy create widespread fear and panic.

In personal relationships, love fades when the other person stops providing enough emotional input and personal attention—those external supports without which the ego falters. When conflicts arise, people suffer in silence or fight futilely to get the other person to change. The ego insists that a better spouse, a bigger house, and more money will bring the satisfaction you long for. What doesn't occur to people is that failing to be satisfied might not be their fault *or* the fault of their circumstances. They might simply have chosen the wrong path to begin with.

The ego's vision of fulfillment is unattainable because each isolated "I" is on its own, cut off from the source of life. The steady improvement being promised can only be external, because there's no security inside. How can there be? The only way the ego can deal with the psyche's disorder and discontent is to wall it off. The "I" is full of secret compartments where fear and anger, regret and jealousy, insecurity and helplessness are forced to hide. Thus we see record levels of anxiety and depression in our society, conditions treated with drugs that just build a thicker wall around the problem. The moment the lulling effect of the drug is removed, depression and anxiety return.

The soul's vision of fulfillment seems far more difficult, and yet it unfolds automatically once you reach the level of the soul. Fulfillment is not a matter of self-improvement. It involves a shift away from the ego's agenda, turning from externals to the inner world. The soul holds out a kind of happiness that isn't dependent on whether conditions outside are good or bad. The path of the soul leads to a place where you experience fulfillment as a birthright, as part of who you are. You don't have to work for it; you only have to be.

Grace comes from a clear vision of who you really are.

Annette's story

Knowing who you really are is the only way to be completely happy. Currently there's a popular notion that travels under the rubric of "stumbling on happiness," the title of a 2006 book by Harvard professor Daniel Gilbert. The core idea is that happiness arrives almost by chance—we stumble on it in the dark, as it were—because people don't really know what will make them happy. This is largely a failure of foresight, Gilbert tells us. We think a million dollars will make us happy, but the day when we actually get a million dollars turns out to be far different from what we saw in advance. The sun doesn't become twice as bright; life doesn't lose its nagging imperfections. If anything, the day you get a million dollars is worse than an ordinary day because it falls so short of being extraordinary.

I have no problem with the observation that people lack the tools to make themselves happy, or with the notion that we rarely see in advance what will actually create happiness. The sentimental image of the sad millionaire is real enough. The most memorable moments of shining happiness do occur unexpectedly. But it's completely wrong, in my view, to assert that human life must be flawed in this way. The deeper truth is that we stumble on identity. We cobble together a self, using the imperfect plans laid down by the ego. We are motivated by memories of what hurt in the past and what felt good, which impel us to repeat the good things and avoid the bad. As a result, "I" is a product of accident, fickle likes and dislikes, old conditioning, and the countless voices of other people who told us what to do and how to be. At bottom, this whole structure is totally unreliable and, in fact, unreal. Having seen through this jerry-rigged self, you should let it go completely. It is the wrong ship to take you to the far shore of fulfillment, and it always was.

"For years I was having a problem in relationships. Basically I never felt loved enough," said Annette, a successful, independent woman I know from teaching a meditation group. "The last man I was involved with only chose me because the woman he wanted to marry got engaged to somebody else. I began to feel that I had never mattered to him at all. So when we broke up, I went to see a therapist.

"She asked me what I wanted to achieve in therapy. That's not an easy question, but I knew that I didn't feel loved, so I told her that I wanted to get over that feeling. The therapist asked me what being loved meant to me. Did I want to be protected, taken care of, coddled? None of those things, I said. To me, being loved means that you are understood. The words just popped out, but they felt right. When I was growing up, nobody understood me at all. My parents were nice people, and they did their best. But their love didn't include understanding who I was. They were too concerned with me finding the right man, making a home together, and raising a family."

"So you started on an inner journey," I said.

Annette nodded. "My therapist turned out to be great. We uncovered all my hidden issues—I kept back nothing. I really trusted her. For months I relived everything about my past. There were lots of revelations and lots of tears."

"But you felt you were achieving something," I said.

"As I released my old stuff, the sense of release was incredible," said Annette. "Before I knew it, five years had passed, hundreds of sessions. One afternoon I was in my therapist's office when it hit me. 'You understand me completely,' I said to her. 'I have no more secrets to tell, no more shameful thoughts and forbidden desires.' At that moment I didn't know whether to laugh or cry."

"Why was that?" I asked.

"Here this woman totally understands me," said Annette. "I have what I've always wanted, and yet what had come of it? I wasn't suddenly happier or more contented. That's what made me want to cry. What made me want to laugh was harder to explain."

"You had come to an end point," I suggested. "That implies the start of a new life."

"I think so. It took a while for it to sink in. But then I noticed that when I'd get in a situation that used to make me angry, instead of flaring up, a voice inside me would say, 'Why are you doing this again? You know where it comes from." The voice was right. I knew myself too well now. Going back to my old reactions wasn't possible."

This proved to be a major turning point. Annette had earned the rare privilege of being able to reexamine herself from the ground up. She had come to the end of everything the ego-self had built up over the years. Once she saw it for what it was—a haphazard, flimsy construct unrelated to her real self—she could move on. Her mind was no longer tied to the past.

The mind can be used for many things, but most people mainly use it as a storehouse. They fill it with memories and experiences, along with all the things they like and dislike. What makes us save some parts of our past and discard others? It's not that we hold on to pleasurable experiences and throw away painful ones. There's a personal attachment to both. Without attachment, the past would simply fade away. I don't mean that you would have amnesia. Attachment is psychological. It preserves the pain that still hurts, and the pleasure that hopes to be repeated. Being in the past, however, your mental storehouse is filled with a jumble of things that no longer serve you.

I said something like this to Annette, and she absolutely agreed. "It had been my fantasy that the real me was hiding out somewhere in my past. If someone wiser and stronger than me was handed all the pieces, they'd hand me back a complete person."

Getting beyond the ego-self means leaving stale illusion behind and beginning to face a fresh reality. We're all clinging to images of ourselves that pile up year after year. Some images make us look good, some make us look bad. But images can't substitute for the real thing. The real you is vital and alive, shifting and changing at every moment. What fascinates me about Annette is that she's one of the few people I've ever met who came to the end of the ego-self. Working with her therapist, she exhausted everything it had to offer. In everyone's life, the ego extends its lease by saying, "Hold on. Keep trying. I know what to do." But stand back and consider what this strategy comes down to:

If all your hard work hasn't brought you what you want, work harder.

If you don't have enough, get more.

If your dream fails, keep following it.

If you grow insecure, believe in yourself more.

Never acknowledge failure; success is the only option.

This kind of ego motivation, turned into slogans, is deeply ingrained in popular culture. Following your dream and never giving up has become a credo repeated by the rich, famous, and successful. Yet for every winner of a beauty pageant, stock-car race, World Series, or Hollywood audition, there are an untold number whose dream didn't come true. They followed their dream just as hard and believed in it just as much. By no means did the ego's strategy work for them. Fortunately, there's another way; it's the exact opposite of the ego's strategy:

> If all your hard work hasn't brought you what you want, look for new inspiration.
>
> If you don't have enough, find it in yourself.
>
> If your dream fails, and you see that it was a fantasy, find a dream that matches your reality.
>
> If you grow insecure, detach yourself from the situation until you find your center again.
>
> You are not shaken by either success or failure; the flow of life brings both, as temporary states.

The real self is a shifting, elusive phantom that's always one step ahead of us. It dissolves the instant you think you're about to grab it. (I've heard God described that way, as someone we constantly run after, only to discover that wherever he—or she—was last seen, he just left.) You can't ever nail down who you really are. To understand your real self, you have to keep up as it moves. Finding the real you happens on the run. The same holds true for grace, since it is part of the real you.

Placing your faith

We have arrived at a point that will be uncomfortable for many people. A fluid, shifting self represents a radical change from the fixed, secure self that the ego promises to provide for us. Feeling the ground beneath your feet suddenly soften is disturbing. Yet the process of letting go leads us to this point. A shift of allegiance is called for. Surrender brings the descent of grace, but not in one flash. Grace is a way of life that relies on none of the ego's old props. Jesus put it succinctly:

> *Do not lay up for yourselves treasures on earth, where moth and rust destroy and where thieves break in and steal; but lay up for yourselves treasures in heaven, where neither moth nor rust destroys and where thieves do not break in and steal.*
>
> (MATTHEW 6:19–20)

Our old way of life centered on saving, planning, looking ahead, providing for security, and relying on material goods must give way to a new one based on trust in Providence, no planning or looking ahead, and nonphysical treasures. The same theme is reiterated throughout the Sermon on the Mount. I said earlier that Saint Paul doesn't provide a process by which grace overtakes a person. The same holds true for Jesus as we meet him in the Gospels. Deep transformation is necessary, yet the steps to get a person from here to there aren't outlined. Instead, Jesus and Paul put the primary emphasis on faith.

Faith is an inner certainty that such radical change can and will happen. But faith needn't be blind. Nor does it have to be based on anything outside yourself. By going through the process of letting go, you will find that there are reasons to have faith here and now.

Faith in your experience. Letting go brings the experience of being tuned in to your soul. As a result, the soul begins to play a bigger role in your life. Gradually but steadily, you begin to have some of the following experiences:

I feel inspired.
I see the truth of spiritual teaching.
I sense that I have a higher self.
A deeper reality is dawning.
My inner life brings satisfaction.

I understand things in a new way.
I greet each day with fresh energy.
My life feels more whole.

Sometimes I tell people to write these things down on a slip of paper to carry around with them. If they can pull out the list and connect with just one item on the list, they are tuned in. If not, then it's time to start tuning in. The flow of life is self-renewing. It brings fresh energy every day to address fresh challenges. But when the soul connection isn't being made, that energy doesn't arise as it should.

Where does faith enter in? When you are aligned with your soul, life feels unbounded, and your awareness exudes carefree joy and confidence. But when you tune out, these qualities disappear. In those moments, have faith in your own experience, which tells you firsthand that being unbounded is real. It's a state of awareness you can return to. I find that the ego-self is like a small, comfortable hut, while what the soul offers is a vast landscape with an infinite horizon. All of us retreat into our hut from time to time. Sometimes we do this under stress, sometimes from pure habit. The psyche is unpredictable enough that you can find yourself feeling insecure for no good reason.

Fortunately, the reason doesn't matter. Once you've experienced freedom, you will be drawn there again. You will find it more comfortable to expand, and as time goes on, the temptation to retreat back into your hut will weaken. There's no need to put pressure on yourself. Freedom speaks for itself; the impulse to experience it is built into you and will never die. That's the first and most important thing to have faith in.

Faith in your knowledge. People who pride themselves on being rational often reject spirituality because it isn't backed up by hard facts. Their argument has a blind spot, however, because not all facts can be measured. It may be a fact that the North Pole is located at 90 degrees north latitude, but it's also a fact that each of us thinks, feels, wishes, and dreams, and upon this invisible reality all external facts depend. The North Pole would have no location without a mind to measure it.

As you walk the path, you acquire knowledge that can be relied upon. Some crucial knowledge has been communicated in these pages, but it's left to you to verify it. What kinds of facts do I have in mind?

Awareness can change the body.

Subtle action can bring you more love and compassion.

Distorted energy patterns can be healed.

The flow of life supplies unlimited energy creativity, and intelligence.

Every problem contains a hidden solution.

Awareness can be either contracted or expanded.

There's another way to live that your ego doesn't know about.

By this point, none of these statements should sound mystical. Even if you feel tentative about one or more of them, have faith that real knowledge does exist in the realm of awareness. The awareness you were born with as a child has expanded over the years. You have added new skills and neural pathways to your brain. Neurologists have confirmed that spiritual practices like meditation are real in physical terms; so is a spiritual attainment like compassion.

Therefore, the process of awakening the soul requires little extra faith. It's a natural extension of findings that have a solid foundation in science. Not that this should be your final proof. I was inspired long ago by a phrase from the French philosopher Jean-Jacques Rousseau: he said that each person was born to test a "soul hypothesis." In other words, you and I are grand experiments, conducted inside ourselves, to prove whether there is a soul. The experiment renews itself in every age. Once it was based on faith in God and scripture. Now it is based on faith that consciousness can grow and evolve. The terms have shifted, but not the challenge.

Faith in yourself. Popular culture constantly drums into us that having faith in yourself leads to the highest achievement. But the self in question really means the ego, with its unquenchable craving to win, own, consume, and find pleasure. That's the last thing to put your faith in. Better to reframe the whole issue as faith in a self you have yet to meet. Nobody needs to have faith in the ego-self; its demands are constant. But the self you have not yet met does require faith, because it is the end point of transformation. Until you undergo this transformation, you are a caterpillar dreaming of turning into a butterfly.

How can you have faith in a self you haven't met? That's such a personal question that the answer will be different for everyone. So let me put the question differently: What would convince you that you have changed at a deep level, and permanently? Here are some answers that most people, I think, would find valid:

I am not in pain anymore.
I don't feel conflicted anymore.
I overcame a weakness and became strong.
Guilt and shame have disappeared.
My mood isn't anxious anymore.
Depression has lifted.
I have found a vision I believe in.
I experience clarity in place of confusion.

These changes are all rooted in the self, because the conditions that need the deepest change—depression, anxiety, conflict, confusion—feel like part of "me." A person doesn't catch them like catching a cold. They may submit to temporary distractions, but the affliction returns. Freud called anxiety an unwelcome visitor who refuses to leave. Every step you take in throwing out an unwelcome visitor is a step of faith in yourself. You are succeeding in letting go. More than that, a new "me" is gradually being revealed. For it turns out that the transformed self isn't like a passenger waiting for the train to arrive. Your new self is revealed one aspect at a time.

Spiritual tradition holds that the soul possesses every virtue. It is beautiful, truthful, strong, loving, wise, understanding, and imbued with the presence of God. Those qualities cannot be taken away. They cannot be bought or acquired by your ego, either, except on a provisional basis. The most loving person can exchange love for hate. The strongest person can be crushed. But as your real self is revealed, all these qualities become unconditional. You won't be aware that they've descended upon you—grace isn't a shower of cool water or white light. Rather, you will simply be yourself. Yet when love is called for, love will be there in you, ready to express itself. When strength is called for, strength will be there. Otherwise, you will feel nothing special. Life goes on as it does for everyone. But inside, in a way hard to describe, you are totally secure. You know that you possess everything you need to confront life's difficulties.

The modern Sufi teacher A. H. Almass expresses this beautifully in an essay titled "Hanging Loose":

> *When your mind is free, not concerned or worried, or focused on anything in particular, and your heart is not grasping or clinging to anything, then you are free. . . . Whatever is there, is there. The mind isn't saying, "I want this" or "I want to look at this" or "It has to be this way." The mind is loose. The expression "hang loose" tells us what it means to be liberated.*

The process of surrender gets you to the point that you can hang loose, without the urge to grab at things and worry over them. The ego's agenda falls away. This takes time, but it comes eventually. Long before that moment, your mind learns what it's like to be quiet, comfortable, and loose. You coast along enjoying this state, and as you do, grace brings in the real you to fill the space once occupied by the mind's churning. To your surprise, you go into a situation where love is called for, and you have that love. It is part of you (just as you suspected in your heart of hearts). In the same inexplicable way, courage has become part of you, and also truth. The promises of the great

spiritual teachers, who told you that grace is freely given, come to fulfillment. Then you know, once and for all, that placing faith in yourself was fully justified. So it must be justified at this moment,
wherever you may be on the journey.

In Your Life: Meeting Grace Halfway

Grace brings about personal transformation, but this happens so quietly that even the most blessed people may not recognize it, or if they
do, they may forget. It's beneficial to put any blessing to work. In that
way it becomes a part of you that goes out into the world. You represent grace through your actions, not as a private possession to be
admired behind closed doors.

If you want to display grace, you need to manifest the qualities of
grace. The words associated with grace in the New Testament provide
a guide:

Merciful
Freely bestowed
Available to all
Generous
Forgiving

I'm not holding these out as moral virtues or as a duty. Rather,
they are a litmus test. You can measure how much grace has come
into your life by the ease with which these actions can be performed.
There's a big difference between giving from the ego and giving from
the soul, between showing mercy and extending forgiveness. The difference can be felt inside, and it's unmistakable.

Showing mercy. Most people show mercy because it's less trouble,
or it makes them feel magnanimous. The ego gets something out of
it, in any event. The image of a condemned man in court comes to
mind. He hangs his head. At that moment the judge holds all the

power, and whether he is harsh or lenient, that power is validated. But the mercy that comes from grace is selfless. You empathize with the wrongdoer. You see his vulnerability and desperation. You understand that more people are changed by an act of mercy than by years of punishment. In short, you see shared humanity in another person, and that requires the eyes of the soul.

Not that mercy must follow the model of a courtroom. You are showing mercy when you don't point out someone else's faults, when you refuse to blame even though blame is deserved, when you refrain from gossiping and bringing someone down behind his back. It's merciful to see the best motives in a person, to give the benefit of the doubt, to look for positive change. In all these instances, you take the nonjudgmental view. Hamlet says, "Use every man after his desert, and who shall escape whipping?" It's a gift of grace not to use every man according to what he deserves, but as mercy pleads.

Bestowing freely. The ego looks out on a world of barter, where everything has a price and quid pro quo is the rule. This doesn't apply to grace. It is given freely, without a thought about what will be given in return. It's unfortunate that the New Testament rests its argument on the sinful nature of man. Saint Paul's notion is that we are all so degraded that we deserve God's wrath and punishment, but, like a loving father, God forgives his errant children. This kind of moral scheme speaks to many people. They feel the weight of their faults and wrongdoing. God becomes the more lovable by overlooking all their sins and erasing them through the power of grace.

There's no need for morality to enter into it, however. It is in the nature of the soul to give freely in the same way that a river gives water. Establish a channel, and the water flows. The ego gets tangled up in questions of who deserves what, calculating how much to give and take away. Grace is free with its gifts. It helps to remember that the universe supplies you with everything, and whether your ego thinks you got enough or not is irrelevant. Your body has been freely sustained with energy, intelligence, and nourishment since the moment of your inception. To the extent that human beings are deprived, the root cause is ultimately ourselves, or our circumstances. It's not in the setup of life that unfolded for billions of years before human beings came on the scene. As freely as one breath comes and the next one goes, you can act from grace by giving without attachment.

Available to all. Grace is the great leveler. It recognizes no differences, but gives itself to anyone who has surrendered. (In Christian metaphor, the rain falls on the just and unjust.) On the other hand, our ego places critical importance on being special. We want someone who loves us more than anyone else in the world. We crave status, recognition, a sense of uniqueness. Yet from the soul's perspective, uniqueness is a universal trait. You are a singular creation no matter what you do; there's no need to prove it to anyone else.

When you make someone feel that he or she is your equal, you exhibit this quality of grace. This holds true whether you are reaching down or reaching up. It's not a question of noblesse oblige, or of giving to the poor because you have so much more. In the eyes of the soul, equality is simply a fact, and you are acknowledging it. When the ego dominates, we all assess where we stand, high or low, in any situation. We are drawn to people who reflect back our own self-image. We subtly put others in their place. Under the influence of grace this behavior changes, because you genuinely feel no higher and no lower than anyone else. A tremendous relief accompanies this realization. So much energy is wasted protecting our dignity, status, pride, and accomplishments. When defending yourself from a fall becomes pointless, you've made an enormous advance toward liberation.

Generous. To be generous is to allow your spirit to overflow. You can be generous at every level of life—giving someone the benefit of your joy is just as good as giving them money, time, or a chance to be heard. Whenever you are generous, you strike a blow against lack. Your ego secretly fears ruin because it believes that something is lacking. This may be the result of scarce resources, an unfair God, bad luck, or personal defect. It's rare to find anyone who doesn't worry, at one time or another, about one or all of these deficiencies. Grace brings living proof that nothing is lacking, either in you or the world around you.

I imagine that there's no wider gap between the ego and the soul than this one. If you declare that there is no lack in the world, countless arguments will be raised against you, and you stand a good chance of being called insensitive, blind, immoral, or worse. Haven't you deliberately overlooked the vast extent of poverty and famine in the world? Jesus' words about Providence watching the fall of a sparrow seem unconvincing to someone who doesn't know where the next meal is coming from. But the teaching is based on consciousness, not on this year's feast or famine. Grace is generous once it has descended, and before that, material forces hold sway.

The ego's generosity is a display of riches; it draws attention to the giver's wealth and the receiver's need. The soul's generosity draws no attention to itself. The impulse is natural and selfless, like a tree loaded with fruit whose branches bow to the ground. If you can be generous from an overflow of spirit, you will be acting from grace.

Showing forgiveness. Here is the most telling test. To forgive unconditionally is a mark of grace. Your ego can't duplicate this quality of the soul. Without grace, forgiveness is always conditional. We wait until we aren't angry anymore. We weigh what is fair and unfair. We nurse grievances and imagine retaliation (or carry it out before we forgive). Conditions are being imposed. When you are able to forgive by setting those conditions aside, you are acting from grace.

Some spiritual teachers would say that the ego can never forgive to begin with. Christianity makes forgiveness a divine attribute. Fallen humanity, itself in severe need of forgiveness, cannot abolish sin without salvation. Buddhism believes that pain and suffering are inherent in human nature until the illusion of the separate self is overcome. It's not that these traditions are pessimistic, or that wrongdoing is a permanent curse. Rather, Jesus and Buddha took a realistic look at the psyche, which is entangled in a complex web of right and wrong. We cannot help but feel that pain is wrong—our own pain, that is— and with that in mind, all wounds are proof of unfairness. Pain makes us feel victimized. Which means that life's tendency to bring pain makes everything and everyone open to blame. If you had to forgive everything you blame someone else for, the process would consume a lifetime.

To extend forgiveness shows that you have found a way out of the trap. Forgiveness becomes easy once you stop being attached to *not* forgiving. The blame game is over. So is the perception of being victimized. In the presence of grace, forgiveness is a recognition that for every wound there is a healing. If you see yourself as healed in advance, there is nothing to forgive in the first place.

Breakthrough #5

The Universe Evolves Through You

Finally, it takes a breakthrough to reveal how precious you really are. Almost no one believes that he or she is absolutely necessary in the grand scheme of things. Yet if you are the growing tip of evolution, the universe needs you in a unique way. You fit into a plan that cannot be imagined in advance. It has no rigid guidelines, no fixed boundaries, and no predictable outcome. The plan is made up as it goes along, and it depends on the participation of each and every person.

I once heard a famous Indian guru talking about the cosmic plan—or the divine plan, as he called it. He couched the plan in the most inspiring terms, painting a future of untold abundance and the total absence of suffering. There was a large audience in attendance, mostly westerners. In the room I could feel an emotional tug-of-war—people wanted to believe what they heard, but they didn't dare. Finally a brave soul stood up and asked, "Is the divine plan unfolding right now? The world looks so chaotic and violent. Fewer and fewer people believe in God."

Without hesitation the guru said, "Belief in God doesn't matter. The plan is eternal. It will always unfold. It can't be stopped." With a sweep of his arm he added, "Everyone here should join. There's no higher purpose in life, and if you join now, you will reap the first rewards."

The questioner's brow furrowed. "What if I don't join?" he asked. "What happens then?"

The guru's face became stern. " The divine plan doesn't need you to unfold." He leaned closer to the microphone. "But if you turn away, it won't unfold through you."

Ultimately, I think that's the right answer. If we take "divine" out of the equation and talk in terms of a universe that is constantly evolving, you can join in the evolutionary flow or not. The choice is yours. Either way, evolution will proceed, but if you opt out, it won't proceed through you.

Why do I matter?

In the past, life was made easier by knowing what God had in store. If you know where you fit in the divine scheme, the physical hardships of life become secondary. If you don't fall in line, your destiny will be painful but no less fixed. I know of no culture in which a person's fate was left adrift. Even in Judaism, where one interpretation (but not all) denies the existence of an afterlife, God dictates that this lifetime, being the only one, should be lived as devoutly as possible. The virtue of living under God is that your small existence has not just a higher purpose, but the highest of all as part of God's creation.

Yet, powerful as it is to live for God, religion has always been vexed by a serious contradiction. Everyone is considered precious to God, but no one is really needed. Individual lives are thrown away in war by the tens of thousands every year. Untold more lives are lost through disease and famine, or barely get a start before infant mortality strikes. Few people talk about this contradiction, yet it has a hidden effect. Doctors must deliver fatal news to patients with incurable conditions. The news comes as a shock, yet it's moving to see that the majority of dying patients are selfless. The reason they don't want to die is that their families need them. The great question "Why am I here?" comes down to other people. This also accounts for the dominant fear expressed by the old, which isn't fear of dying or even of chronic, disabling pain. Rather, old people are most afraid that they will become a burden to their children.

It's only human to realize that we all need each other. But if taken too far, this becomes a system of codependency in the worst sense: I only exist to need and be needed. I remember, early in my medical training, wishing that just one person, upon hearing that he had incurable liver or pancreatic cancer, would murmur, "What a loss to the world when I am gone." Not a loss to one's family and friends but an absolute loss, something that makes the world poorer. We see the passing of eminent people that way, certainly. Yet from your soul's perspective, you are as great an addition to the world as Mahatma Gandhi or Mother Teresa, and subtracting you from the cosmic equation would be just as great a loss. The most exquisite silk remains intact if you pull out a thread, but the snag will show.

Many people would resist the notion that they have an absolute worth in the universe. Unwittingly they are playing out a behavior known as learned helplessness. A famous example comes from experiments on dogs performed in the 1950s. Two dogs were put in separate cages, and each was given a mild shock at random intervals. The first dog had a switch that it could hit to make the shocks stop, and very quickly it learned to throw the switch. Since the shocks were mild, this dog displayed no adverse effects. The second dog received shocks at the same time, but had no switch for stopping them. Its experience was very different. For that dog, pain was a random occurrence out of its control.

But it's the second part of the experiment that is most revealing. Each dog was now put into a cage where half the floor delivered shocks while the other half was safe. All the dog had to do when it was shocked was to jump over a small partition to reach the safe zone. The first dog, the one that had learned how to turn the shocks off, didn't have a switch anymore. But it didn't need one. It quickly learned to jump to safety. The second dog, however, gave up immediately. It lay down and let the shocks come as they would, without making an effort to jump out of the way. This is learned helplessness in action. When applied to human life, the implications are devastating. Countless people accept that life's pain and suffering come randomly. They have never been in control of the shocks that every existence delivers, and so they seek no escape, even when one is presented.

Knowing how things work is important. Otherwise, learned

helplessness creeps up on us. The first dog learned that life makes sense: if you hit a switch, the pain goes away. The second dog learned that life was pointless: no matter what you do, the pain comes anyway, which means either no one is in charge, or whoever's in charge doesn't care. A dog's brain may not think this way, but ours do. Without a sense of purpose, we resort to helplessness, since either God isn't there or he doesn't care what happens to us. To escape our learned helplessness, we have to have a sense that we matter in the larger scheme of things.

Brett's story

Our purpose is hidden from us, yet there are moments when we see that everything fits together. We may not know what the plan is, but for certain we know that *something* is working out a larger design; at such times we realize that the most common events cohere into extraordinary patterns.

At seventy, Brett is an avid gardener. One rose in his garden is tall and strikingly beautiful, its blooms pale yellow tinged with pink. "This is the only mystical rose I grow, and it has a story," he told me. "When the Nazis invaded France, flower-growing came to a sudden halt. Every available acre had to be used for food, so a young grower near Lyon found himself digging up 200,000 rosebushes to be burned. He was an avid breeder; it crushed him to destroy the decades of work started by his father and grandfather, so he saved his most promising seedling. The war grew darker, and he was lucky enough to send a package containing buds of this new rose to America with one of the last diplomatic couriers leaving France.

"He had no idea what happened to this handful of bud grafts until France was liberated in 1944. Within weeks he got an excited telegram. The rose had thrived overseas, and it wasn't just promising. It was stupendous, perhaps the greatest rose the American nurseries had ever seen. It was decided to set a date, at which point the public would be introduced to 'Peace,' as the rose would be called. A series of coincidences followed that became legend. When the naming day came, it coincided with the day that Japan surrendered. On the day that 'Peace' won the award for best rose of the year 1945, Germany surrendered. On the day that the first delegates gathered to form the United Nations, each was greeted with a blossom of 'Peace.' As it turned out, this was also the day that Germany signed the final papers of surrender."

Brett paused. "Everyone in the rose world knows about 'Peace,' which became by far the most famous rose in the world. It sold in the millions. It made a fortune for the young French grower, whose name was Francis Meilland. But that's not why I call this rose mystical. It was Meilland's tragedy to die young, at the age of forty-six. Before he passed away, he visited his oncologist, and on a table in the waiting room was placed a bowl of 'Peace,' which seems like little more than a coincidence. But when Meilland returned home, he told his family that he saw his mother sitting next to the roses, smiling at him. She had passed away twenty years before, and in her honor, her son had given 'Peace' another name in France, 'Madame Antoine Meilland.' What do you think of that?"

I could see that this story was emotional for Brett. "What do *you* think of it?" I asked.

"I think it was preordained, the whole thing. As if the first seed, which Meilland planted in 1935, was meant to become a symbol for world peace after the war. People took it that way. Who's to deny them?"

"I guess you could say that official reality denies them," I pointed out. "A string of coincidences is just that."

"I know," said Brett. "You have to be naïve or fanciful to think that everything could fit together so perfectly. It's as if each event knew that it was part of the same story, and we can't have that, can we?"

It depends. Many people casually say that "nothing happens without a reason." Yet at the same time they don't see an overarching purpose to their lives. Animals are free from this dilemma. You can see their purpose simply by observing it. A hungry cow eats; a cat in heat mates. Human purpose, however, is rarely visible. When you see a crush of Christmas shoppers jamming the stores, all are doing the same thing, but they don't share the same purpose. Some are full of holiday spirit and want to give pleasure with their gifts. Others are carrying out a social ritual. Still others are addicted consumers.

It would help a great deal to know what the overall plan is. Otherwise we are left to observe a collection of individuals, each of whom is groping for purpose and catching glimpses of it far too rarely.

The rules of the game

The plan for the unfolding universe stands right before us, even though we fail to see it. We're blind to it because the plan *is us*. Or, to make it personal, you are the cosmic plan—or the divine plan, if you prefer. There are no rules outside your mind, no actions outside your body. Whatever you choose to do, the plan bends to accommodate. When you have a new desire, the universe shifts accordingly. It has no choice, because there is no purpose to creation beyond you, right here and right now.

I know that this description sounds like hyperbole. All your life you have absorbed a worldview that puts you under a higher power. If it isn't the power of God, it's the power of natural forces. If it isn't the power of authority figures, it's the power of human nature and its self-destructive impulses. None of that is true—or, to be precise, none of that is true once you discover your real self. Ultimately, to discover your purpose comes down to discovering who you really are.

The cosmic plan that was built into you follows certain invisible guidelines:

1. *Everything is conscious.* There are no dead zones in creation. Consciousness is an activity of the entire universe, which

means that when you are aware of anything, the universe is aware through you. What you see and do alters the whole scheme.

2. *Everything fits together.* There are no loose parts to the universe, nothing is left over. Wholeness keeps each part in place and assigns each its necessary role. When anything looks random, you are seeing one pattern moving into another.

3. *The whole scheme is self-organizing.* No outside controller is needed. Once a galaxy, a butterfly, a heart, or an entire species is on the move, its inner workings know what to do.

4. *Evolution unfolds within itself.* Once something grows, it seeks the highest form of itself—the best star, dinosaur, fern, or amoeba. When that form is exhausted, it makes a transition to a new form that is more creative and interesting.

5. *Freedom is the ultimate goal.* You don't win by getting to the end; you win by finding a new game the instant the old one is over. This isn't an empty freedom. You never find yourself floating in a void. Rather, this is the freedom of possibilities that never run out.

At every level, Nature follows these five guidelines. They are invisible; they exist only in consciousness. The reason you haven't been aware of them isn't God's secrecy. The plan isn't abstract. Quite the opposite—it's built into every cell in your body. You can become aware of the plan if you choose, and then the universe acquires a new face.

1. *Everything is conscious.* Living in accord with this truth means that you respect all life forms. You believe that you are a part of a living whole, and you act as if all your actions help the whole to evolve. You recognize a kinship with every level of consciousness, from the lowest to the highest.

2. *Everything fits together.* This truth opens your mind to see how the whole of life interacts. Instead of thinking in

mechanical terms, you see each event unfolding organically. Instead of taking life one piece at a time, you look for the larger picture. It would also be natural to investigate how and why things fit together. Is there an overarching intelligence that is thinking on the cosmic scale? If so, then are you a thought in this universal mind, or part of the thinking process—or both?

3. *The whole scheme is self-organizing.* This is one of the most fascinating truths, because it holds that nothing has a beginning or an end. The universe isn't like the tide going in and out again. It's like the ocean as a whole, breathing in and out, sending up waves that fall back again into the wholeness. No event is separate. We only see separateness because our perspective is narrow. Through a wider lens you can see that all events arise together.

    Think of an ant that has learned to read. It is the world's most intelligent ant, but it's still quite small, so it reads a book by crawling from one word to the next. The plot of the book is completely linear from the ant's perspective, so it would be amazed to know that you—a much bigger creature—can approach the book as a whole, and you can dip into it wherever you want, read the end before the beginning, sample high spots, or select only what interests you. You can do all those things because the linear is only one mode of many in approaching a book. The same is true of life.

4. *Evolution unfolds within itself.* Once you see that linear thinking is just a choice—and a fairly arbitrary one—you can look at evolution in a new way. Think of that museum diagram showing a stooped-over primate turning into a Neanderthal, then a caveman and finally *Homo sapiens*, each one standing taller and straighter. That's a perfect example

of linear thinking, but it overlooks that the driving force of human evolution is the brain, and it didn't develop in a straight line, not even remotely. It grew in a global fashion. Every new area of the brain added to the evolution of the whole. Every new skill was recognized by the whole brain.

For example, when our ancestors first stood upright, this affected motor coordination, eyesight, balance, blood circulation, and many other aspects of the body-mind you recognize as your own. The opposable thumb, offered as a textbook example of physical evolution that separates human beings from lower primates, would be meaningless without a brain that learned the infinite possibilities inherent in this new ability to press a thumb against a forefinger. It took a global response by the brain to develop from this rudimentary skill all of art, agriculture, tools, buildings, and weapons. Evolution is a total activity of the universe.

5. *Freedom is the ultimate goal.* If evolution is happening everywhere in a global fashion, where is it heading? For centuries human beings assumed that we were the highest goal of God's creation, and despite Darwin's shocking demotion of humans to one species among many, we still believe we hold a privileged place. But it's not at the top of the ladder of life. Instead, we are the one creature who grasps that creativity is infinite. Evolution is heading everywhere, not to an end point. The ultimate goal of the universe is to unfold without limits. To put it in a word, evolution is becoming more and more free, and its ultimate goal is total freedom.

Laws of nature dictate how units of matter combine when atom collides with atom, yet infinite variety is permitted at the same time. We are embedded in a design that is dynamic, free, creative, and unpredictable. Evidence of this lies in what we call games. Consider how a baseball game is run. It exists entirely in consciousness. Human beings decided that hitting a leather ball with a stick has value. Invisible rules were devised that each player keeps in his head. No one speaks of these rules as the game is being played, but infractions are instantly noticed and penalized. The baseball field is strictly demarked with lines and boundaries, yet within these limits the players are free to improvise. No two games are exactly alike; no two players have the same style, or level of talent. And once a game starts, this combination of fixed rules and free play determines who wins. A baseball game is open-ended until the bottom of the ninth inning, despite the rigid set of rules that enclose it.

Every game is a display of consciousness in creative mode. The universe is in the same mode. The defenders of so-called intelligent design—the notion that an all-knowing Creator made everything in the universe to fit perfectly—aren't wrong to stand in awe before creation. The real problem is that intelligent design isn't intelligent enough. It limits God to one big idea that never changes, when in reality the universe changes constantly and is ever more inventive.

If the whole universe is conscious, we have an instant explanation for why nothing is accidental. Yet it's hard to imagine a rock by the side of the road being as conscious as you and I are. There's a way to get past this objection, however. Imagine that you live in a dream, but don't know it. Inside your dream you see other people moving around, so they seem conscious to you. You view animals behaving as if they possessed consciousness as well—they are curious, for example, and can be trained into new behavior. But when it comes to rocks and clouds, they are inanimate, so you assume they aren't conscious. Then someone comes along and says, "Everything is conscious. It has to be. All that you see around you is happening in a person's brain. That person is you. You are the dreamer, and as long as this is your dream, it shares in your consciousness."

There is only the finest line between "I am dreaming" and "I am in a dream," since the brain creates both states. Why not cross the line? In some cultures, no other invitation is needed. The ancient rishis of India compared life to a dream because all experience is subjective. There is no way to experience the world except subjectively. If every experience happens "in here," it makes perfect sense that things all fit together: we make them fit together. Even randomness is a concept created by the human brain. As mosquitoes swarm at sunset, they don't feel random, nor do atoms of interstellar dust. We don't see form and design until they fit our preconceptions, but this doesn't matter to Nature. Seem through an electron microscope, every cell in your body looks like a swirling haze of activity, but that's just a perception. As far as Nature is concerned, every aspect of your body is orderly and purposeful.

So you face a choice. You can take the position that order only exists where humans say it does, or you can take the position that order is everywhere. Either way, all you've done is to take a point of view. If half the people in the world said that God designed all of creation and the other half said that creation was a random event, the universe would still be what it is. Consciousness would still be flowing through your body, brain, mind, and all living creatures, ignoring the artificial boundaries we impose. The either/or isn't between science and religion, but between participating in the cosmic plan or not. There's a voluntary aspect and an involuntary aspect. As with a baseball game, you have to want to play, but once you do, you're all in.

In Your Life: Core Participation

As with any game, once you're in the game of life, you should play to win. You must commit yourself from your very core. Knowing the guidelines of the divine plan gives you an enormous advantage in this regard. Not knowing them is like playing a game whose rules are revealed one at a time, and only when you break them. Life works that way for most people. They discover how to live by trial and error. Other people fall back upon a rule book that is supposed to apply to everyone and cover all contingencies—the Bible is such a rule book, but many others exist. In India, these guides for living (gathered in texts known as the *Puranas*) run to thousands of pages, with minute descriptions of the most arcane situations and combinations of behavior. In the end, however, no one has ever led an exemplary life by following a recipe.

Between having no rules and imposing rigid ones, the universe has left room for dynamic guidelines that impose the least restraint on free will. To participate fully, each guideline allows for maximum achievement. Achievement doesn't mean material success. It means fully understanding how consciousness works.

Your Best Game

Let consciousness do the work.

Don't interfere with the flow.

View everyone as an extension of yourself.

Watch for change and use it wisely.

Gather information from every source.

Wait until your intention is clear.

Realize that nothing is personal—the universe is acting through you.

Ask for nothing less than inspiration.

See every step as part of the process.

These tactics have one thing in common: they are in accord with the invisible plan that underlies everyone's life. But because participation is voluntary, there's a sharp contrast between people who align themselves with the plan and those who don't. Let me illustrate this point by point.

Let consciousness do the work. People who follow this guideline are highly subjective, but their subjectivity isn't fickle; they don't give in to each passing mood. Instead they are self-aware, which means that they know when they are uncomfortable in a situation, and don't move forward until it feels right. Their bodies give them signals of stress and strain that they take seriously. Such people trust themselves, which is a totally subjective state, yet a very powerful one. To trust a self that is rooted in ego would be folly, but when you truly know who you are, you can trust yourself from the soul level. At that level, consciousness isn't merely subjective. It flows through the universe, the soul, the mind, and the body. Letting consciousness do the work means surrendering to an organizing principle that is vaster than yourself, vast enough to keep all of reality together.

Don't interfere with the flow. There is a profound Buddhist doctrine that speaks of a great river that flows through all of reality. Once you have found yourself, there is no more cause for action. The river picks you up and carries you along forever after. In other words, effort from the personal level, the kind of effort all of us are used to in daily life, becomes pointless after a certain point. This includes mental effort. Once you become self-aware, you realize that the flow of life needs no analysis or control, because it's all you. The great river only seems to pick you up. Actually, you have picked yourself up—not as an isolated person, but as a phenomenon of the cosmos. No one gave you the job of steering the river. You can enjoy the ride and observe the scenery.

Learning to step aside from your false responsibilities means giving up your urge to control, defend, protect, and insure against risk. All of that is false responsibility. To the extent that you can let it go, you will stop interfering with the flow. To the extent that you cling, life will continue to bring even more things to control, and to defend yourself against. Risks will loom everywhere. It's not that fate is set against you. You are simply seeing reflections of your deepest beliefs, as consciousness unfolds the drama drawn up beforehand in your mind. It's the universe's task to unfold reality; yours is only to plant the seed.

View everyone as an extension of yourself. When people get on the spiritual path, they often find themselves misunderstood. The accusation is leveled against them (if only behind their backs) that they have become self-centered. The implication is "It's not all about you." If "you" means the isolated ego, that's certainly true. But at the level of the soul, the self changes. Losing its boundaries, it merges with the flow of life. On the spiritual path you come to sense the flow and willingly join it. Then—and only then—is everyone else an extension of yourself. How do you know that you have reached this point? First, you have no enemies. Second, you feel another's pain as your own. Third, you find that a common sympathy links everyone.

As these three perceptions dawn, reality is shifting. You are claiming your new home in the unlimited landscape of spirit. But even before that comes to fruition, you are connected to everyone else. Nothing keeps you from living that truth. There will always be differences of personality. What changes is self-interest. Instead of being about "me," it starts to be about "us," the collective consciousness that binds everyone. On a practical basis this means seeking agreement, consensus, and reconciliation. These are the primary goals for anyone who lives in the flow.

Watch for change and use it wisely. You can use the transient nature of life to your advantage. Most people fear change; others allow it to pass them by. To use change creatively, those attitudes won't work. Nothing will work as a life strategy that isn't dynamic and growing. Change itself is neutral, since for every constructive change there is a destructive one. But the *principle* of change holds the key, for it dictates that going with the flow of life brings growth and creativity, while attempting to freeze events, memories, pleasure, and inspiration brings stasis. The most inspiring or pleasurable moments in your life beg to be savored and held on to. You must resist that temptation, because the minute you try to hang on to an experience, it loses the vitality that made it special in the first place.

Use the principle of change to keep your life fresh and renewable. Taking the attitude that the flow of life is always self-renewing will help you avoid stagnation, and anxiety over the future. What makes people anxious about the future is a gnawing fear that the best has already happened, or that a single missed opportunity will prove to be decisive. "The one that got away" is a recurrent theme of failed romance, and it applies equally to failed careers, abandoned projects, and deflated aspirations. But in reality "the one that got away" comes down to clinging to a fixed idea. Every creative person's success is based on trust that inspiration is continuous. The more you create, the more there is to create. In a documentary on a famous orchestra conductor who was turning eighty, the most poignant moment came with his last comment: "I have no wish to live many more years, except for knowing that I am just beginning to say all that I want to say through my music."

Gather information from every source. The universe is multidimensional, and when we speak of the flow of life, it's a multidimensional flow. Imagine not just one mighty river rushing to the sea, but a hundred small streams converging, mixing, and each adding its unique contribution. To draw the most from life, you must be aware that absolutely anything can contribute to it. Inspiration comes from all directions, both inner and outer. You need alert antennae to sense how continuously your soul is communicating with you. It's not a matter of tuning in to a hundred cable TV channels in the hope of finding one interesting program. Rather, in the welter of sensations that bombard the brain every day, certain ones are meant for you— they carry a meaning that is personal to you alone.

In the Indian tradition it is said that God spends as much time hiding as revealing himself, which points to an everyday truth. The next thing that will spur you on is asleep until you awaken it. The future is a hiding place we call the unknown. Yet the known, which is here and now, comes from nowhere if not from the unknown. The instinct that says "something is out there waiting" is valid. You stand at the pivot point between the unknown and the known. Your task is to reach into the darkness and pluck out the next thing that will be meaningful.

Some people avoid the task by repeating the known over and over. What they don't realize is that the unknown is never truly invisible. Your soul anticipates what you need, and it lays out hints and clues on your path. This is the soul's subtle form of guidance. It winnows out the useless, the pointless, the misleading, and the false starts. If you tune in with alertness, you'll feel a sense of vibrancy

about the thing you should be doing—it feels right, alluring, seduc-
tive, enticing, pleasurable, curious, intriguing, and challenging, all at
once. Being open to those feelings, which are entirely subjective,
allows you to pick up the hints left by your soul. The unknown looks
dark only to those who can't see its hidden glow.

Wait until your intention is clear. Countless people are looking for
motivation in the wrong places. They seek to increase their energy
and drive. They want the biggest reward. They lie in wait for a lightning bolt to hit them with the next great invention or business
idea. The real source of motivation isn't any of those things. Motivation, the kind that carries seed ideas to fruition with energy and passion, comes from a clear intent. Knowing exactly what you want to
do, with unwavering conviction, is the spark that generates everything else, including the big ideas and the great rewards. Confusion
and uncertainty divide the flow of life into separate, weak channels.
Because a clear intent can't be forced, many people never find one.
They apply a bit of themselves to half a dozen areas of their lives. Yet
there is no great secret to finding a clear intent; it depends upon simply waiting.

Waiting isn't a passive act; it only looks passive. The right kind of
waiting involves discrimination: you are inwardly sorting out what
feels right from what doesn't. You allow vague fantasies and idealistic
schemes to do what they will—the pointless ones dissolve in time. You
keep an eye out for a spark that refuses to be extinguished. Much else
is involved—anxious searching, the struggle of self-doubt, the lure of
grandiose ambitions, and flights of impossible fancy. Eventually a clear
intent will emerge, and once it does, the invisible forces harbored in
the soul will come to your aid. For many people, waiting for a clear
intent is so exhausting that they undertake it only a few times, generally in those uncertain years when young adults feel compelled to start
a career. Casting about, they feel aimless and under pressure; they
watch as their more motivated peers pass them by in the job market.

But with hindsight, one can see that the individuals who held
out until a clear intent revealed itself were the lucky ones. Despite

stress, peer pressure, and doubt, they had the inner strength to trust that "something is out there waiting." Or in here waiting. It amounts to the same thing, a hidden potential that needed to be carefully plucked out from the tangled fabric of the psyche. The best thing you can do is to go through this process as many times as possible. The fog that shrouds your soul may be thick, but it will clear if you want it to, however long the process takes.

Realize that nothing is personal—the universe is acting through you. It sounds strange to hear that you shouldn't take your life personally. What could be more personal? Yet the universe's plan is composed entirely of impersonal forces. They apply equally to every object, every event. They are not loaded against you or for you, any more than gravity is. Finding your soul is the same as finding the impersonal self, because the soul has direct access to the invisible forces that uphold the cosmos. Intelligence is impersonal, and so are creativity and evolution. They are discovered only in your deepest awareness. To take full advantage of them, look upon life as a school, with consciousness as its curriculum.

The ego takes everything personally, which is a big hindrance; experience is happening to "me." Buddhism spends a great deal of time trying to dispel the notion that this "me" has a claim on experience. Instead, Buddhists say, the experience is unfolding on its own, and you, as an experiencer, are simply a conduit. Thus we get formulations like "Thinking is thinking itself." It can be baffling to unravel the complexities of such a simple statement as "Being is," or "The dancer is the dance." Yet the essential point is practical: the less you take life personally, the more easily it can flow through you. Holding on lightly works. Holding on tightly doesn't work. Nor does assuming that every experience either builds you up or tears you down. The flow of life doesn't sort itself into plus and minus columns. Everything has its own intrinsic value, measured in energy, creativity, intelligence, and love. To find those values, a person must stop asking, "What good does it do me?" Instead, you witness what happens, finding fascination in all of it.

Ask for nothing less than inspiration. Daily life can be maddeningly mundane. You can overcome the tedium by piling up as many interests as possible, but in the end you may find that you never got below the surface. For what makes life mundane is shallowness. In the depths, every experience is full of vitality. You feel vibrant, no matter what your life looks like on the surface. In some spiritual traditions, making your daily routine vibrant is an ultimate goal. The idea is that you can carry water and chop wood while still feeling universal. I respect those traditions, but sometimes I miss the most vibrant quality that life can offer, which is inspiration. It limits the soul to ask it to fill daily routine with light. Why not fill extraordinary achievement with light?

Consciousness is value-free. It can be shaped into ugly, dull, inert things if your intention moves that way. Like an artist's palette, which is full of colors but which carries no guarantee that lovely pictures will result, consciousness contains vibrancy, brilliance, and fascination. But even a self-aware person doesn't automatically gets a life with those qualities. You must shape consciousness with intent, which is why asking for inspiration is crucial. So is not settling for less. I said before that your soul places hints along the path, clues to the next thing that will spur you on. To be more precise, these hints depend on where you're going and where you're coming from. If you are walking a path of low expectations, the next thing you find will support those low expectations.

Your soul has no agenda. It's not out to make you the best you can be. It's out to fulfill the potential you discover in yourself, which means that you and your soul are in a cooperative venture. You ask, it supplies. What it supplies leads you to ask for the next thing. Because it's rare to meet every occasion with a clear intention, often we ask for things that are mixed up, conflicted, and confused. And when we do, the soul winds up providing us with less-than-ideal opportunities. We find ourselves at loose ends or following false trails. To keep this from happening, ask for nothing less than inspiration. That is to say, keep your highest vision in mind, and in any situation, seek the highest outcome according to that vision.

As always, this strategy is purely subjective; it happens inside.

But only by cleaving steadily to your vision can you align yourself with the highest potential you were born to express. The best you can be comes down to a series of decisions that refuses the less-than-best time and again. We aren't speaking of consumer shopping here. It's not the less-than-best lover, car, house, or job. You refuse the less-than-best idea, motivation, purpose, solution, and goal, choosing instead to wait for better, and trusting that your soul will bring it.

See every step as part of the process. When some people say, "It's all part of the process," one hears a note of resignation, as if life takes time and patience, but if you can put up with the bother long enough, the process eventually works. This makes the process sound like a bureaucracy grinding its way to action, or a conveyor belt that mechanically produces results. The process I'm describing is not like that at all. It is dynamic, unpredictable, fascinating, and ever-changing. To be caught up in the process brings ultimate joy and fulfillment. The great spiritual guides, those who can look at life metaphysically, often declare that the process takes care of itself. A noted Indian guru was once asked, "Is my personal evolution something I'm doing or something that's happening to me?" His answer: "It's both, but if we must choose, it's something that is happening to you."

Yet, for all that, the spiritual path doesn't feel automatic. Here and now, from the ant's perspective rather than that of the eagle, life takes participation. You must focus on every minute; new challenges show up constantly and cannot be ignored. It's all too easy, then, to view your life as a sequence of moments, steps forward or backward. Most people participate in their lives exactly that way, by "living one day at a time," as the saying goes. This perspective would turn all of us into survivors. It would deny life its wholeness, and if you take that away, wholehearted participation is impossible. Of course you will accept one slice of bread at a time if you don't know that the whole loaf can be yours.

We are forced to speak in metaphors because the process of life is mysterious. Does it happen right now if right now you are filling your car with gas, changing a baby diaper, or sitting in the dentist's chair?

Does it unfold to a glorious conclusion on a date you can circle on your calendar? The mingling of the visible and invisible, the sublime and the distressing, is inescapable. The only viable attitude you can take is "This is it." Sometimes "it" amounts to nothing; you can't wait for it to end. Sometimes "it" feels as if the heavens have parted; you can only hope it will last forever. But "it" is a bird on the wing. You'll never catch it. The miracle is that the greatest creations, such as the human brain, were made by chasing after the bird. We weave ourselves into a tapestry of experience that grows more exalted as time passes, yet each thread is nothing but a wisp of thought, desire, or feeling. Every moment lived adds another stitch, and even if you cannot envision what the final pattern will look like, it helps to know that the thread is golden.

1O STEPS TO WHOLENESS

PROMISES YOU
CAN KEEP

Wholeness is the result of connecting body, mind, and soul. In wholeness you aren't divided against yourself; therefore the choices you make are beneficial at every level. Once you realize how the soul functions, there is no reason to turn back and live any other way than from the level of the soul. Yet living without the soul has also been easy. You can ignore being divided against yourself. Life goes on without resolving that issue. Bad decisions bring pain and suffering, but people learn to put up with it. In other words, life without being whole is "easy" because of habit, inertia, or old conditioning that is hard to break. (I remember my first meditation instructor, who insisted that if I wasn't committed to daily practice, I might as well not start. "I don't know how many years it takes to reach enlightenment," he said, "but it takes only one day to quit.")

The secret is to live in wholeness now, before you completely achieve it. What's needed is a lifestyle that keeps your vision alive. "Holistic" has come to mean organic food, leaving no carbon footprint, practicing prevention, and trusting in alternative medicine. All of those things are undeniably good—they are evidence of growing consciousness that earlier generations only dreamed of—but they won't keep you on the spiritual path. A holistic lifestyle should sustain the ties to your soul even when those ties feel fragile.

Spiritual teachers have wrestled with this problem for centuries, wondering how they can bridge the gulf between the old life and the new. Teaching and preaching aren't enough. Showing by example isn't enough. Yet many human beings have crossed over to the light (call them saints, yogis, bodhisattvas, or simply inspiring examples) and what they have achieved is real. If we distill their stories, a lifestyle emerges that applies to you and me in these times of transition. The lifestyle is simple, and can be followed without anyone else needing to know or approve. I've broken it down into simple steps.

10 Steps to Wholeness

1.   Nourish your "light body."
2.   Turn entropy into evolution.
3.   Commit yourself to deeper awareness.
4.   Be generous of spirit.
5.   Focus on relationships instead of consumption.
6.   Relate to your body consciously.
7.   Embrace every day as a new world.
8.   Let the timeless be in charge of time.
9.   Feel the world instead of trying to understand it.
10.   Seek after your own mystery.

These steps happen in awareness. They mean the most to me personally, because they are the fruit of my own journey. As a child in India I learned that my fate hung in the balance between *vidya*, or wisdom, and *avidya*, or ignorance. This choice, which goes back thousands of years, was painted in graphic terms that a young boy could understand. I was born in a time of turmoil as the country was struggling with every imaginable woe, from riots in the streets between Hindus and Muslims to gross social inequity and millions living on the verge of famine. What would save us? Not belief in God or massive social programs, good as those things might be. I was

taught that life followed from the values you held in your own awareness. The road of light, or the road of darkness? By the time I was
eight I knew which one to choose. Happiness, success, prosperity, and
well-being would come my way if I lived by the light of *vidya*.

In later years I lost my innocence and came to see this promise as
somewhat empty, like Benjamin Franklin's promise that "early to bed,
early to rise, makes a man healthy, wealthy, and wise." More effective
was the fear of living in *avidya*, which brought disease, poverty, and
disgrace. These threats were not pumped into me, the way children
are warned that the devil is waiting if they stray from God. Yet for
nearly forty years I wandered between the two poles of wisdom and
ignorance, or, if you will, belief and unbelief. I know firsthand the gap
between vision and reality. Today, as firmly as I believe in self-
transformation, I come back to that gap. Most people know what's
supposed to be good for them, but making promises to themselves ("I
will never cheat," "I won't wind up getting a divorce," "I'll never stab
anyone in the back to get ahead") is never quite enough. (A guru was
once asked by a confused disciple, "Master, how can I become a good
person?" The guru said, "It's nearly impossible. If you think deeply,
there are a thousand reasons to pick a pin up from the floor and a
thousand reasons not to." The disciple became very worried. "Then
what can I do?" The guru smiled. "Find God." Now the disciple was
much more worried. "But, sir, finding God seems so far beyond my
reach." The guru shook his head. "Finding God is a hundred times
easier than trying to be good. God is part of you, and once you locate
that part, being good comes naturally.")

If the spiritual path is to take us to our goal, we must make
promises that we can keep every day. The ten steps I've outlined are
just that. They don't require you to stretch beyond your limits, and
yet your limits will begin to expand. The ten steps can't be under-
mined by old habits and conditioning, because you won't be asked to
fight against your old self. All you can do is help the new self to grow
in silence. Yet nothing more is needed. The secret is that inner transformation cannot be seen as it occurs. The brain shifts as the person

shifts. The brain has no way of preserving its old pathways once new ones have been created. In a sense the soul erases its tracks, and yet something very tangible is also happening.

A good friend was a committed seeker for years. To all outward appearances he led an ordinary life. Whenever I ran into him, I'd ask how his search was going. His reply, offered with a smile, was always the same. "I'm almost ready to peek out of the incubator." This went on for several years. He was very private, and I doubt there were more than a handful of people who knew about his inner dedication. Then the day came when he gave up his strict spiritual disciplines, and he seemed much happier for it. When I asked what had changed, he spoke eloquently.

"When I started out, I was shy about my spirituality. My family thought of me as antireligious, in fact, since I had refused to go to church with them when I turned eighteen. After I started meditating, I thought I was changing, but if anyone saw this, they had nothing to say. People liked the way I used to be. So I quietly kept on, and I let everyone suppose that I was the person I had always been.

"Then I found that my desires weren't the same anymore. There was nothing I desperately wanted or didn't want. I stopped running after the things everyone else thought were so important. My friends and family noticed that I had gotten a lot quieter. That's all they said. I kept working on myself and moved on.

"Time passed, and more changes happened. I faced my ego and its whole deal. I went into my old beliefs and my need to be right all the time. There was something new to look at every day. I kept watching and moving on. Nothing outward was drastically different, but there were moments when I was amazed that the people close to me didn't see how totally different I had become."

"This was all happening while you were in the incubator?" I asked.

My friend smiled. "Exactly. Then one day it all ended. I woke up and had no desire to meditate. Frankly, I felt kind of blank, as if nothing had happened for the last ten years. I looked at myself in the mirror, and this ordinary guy stared back at me. For a second I was almost afraid, feeling a faint wave of dread. I lay back down on the bed, and then, like a warm liquid inside, I felt "it" wash over me. What is "it"? Life itself, like a river picking me up and carrying me along. Since then, I've been going where the river goes, and things just work out. From that moment on, *everything* works out."

His face showed a flush that was a kind of ecstasy. But I had a question. "Why not let the river carry you beginning the first day? Why do you have to wait until the end?"

"That's the thing," my friend said. "I had a thousand days I thought *were* the end. And I'm not sure I could tell you when the first day was, either. The thing happens when it wants to."

In all honesty, none of us knows when the first day on the path was—or when the last day will be. Therefore, the best thing is to live every day as if it were the first *and* the last. A new world is born in spirit every time the sun rises. Life is perpetually fresh, so your path can be just as fresh. Otherwise, if you postpone your life waiting for a great and glorious gift to be bestowed, the gift may never come, and your life will be postponed forever. Wholeness must be seized at this moment, because eternity dawns only in a moment like this one. The goal of the following steps is to make wholeness a daily possibility. Vision and reality want to come together. The time to make that happen is now.

Step 1. Nourish Your "Light Body"

Your soul acts as your spiritual body. As such, it needs to be nourished. In the same way that your cells exchange oxygen and food, your spirit body sends and receives subtle energy, or "light." Your heart, liver, brain, and lungs—all your organs—literally survive on light coming from the sun. Every bite of food represents trapped sunlight that your body releases into chemical and electrical energy. Your cells have no future except through light.

"Light" performs the same function at a subtler level. Every message from your soul is encoded in energy, because the brain must convert love, truth, beauty—every aspect of meaning, in fact—into physical activity. Subtle energy brings the mind into material existence, so in practical terms your future depends on how well you nourish your light body. If you feed it with fresh energy every day, it will provide you with inspiration and guidance. In the West we aren't used to thinking that way, but in Sanskrit the word *jyoti*, or light, is more than physical. *Jyoti* carries meaning, growth, good and bad influences, and the whole trajectory that a person's life will follow. Even if you are a strict materialist and believe that the brain is the source of the mind, nothing is possible in the brain without energy; therefore you wind up with the same conclusion, that a person's hopes, wishes, and dreams must be nourished through light—in this case, sunlight. And you will have to account for how raw light, composed of photons, manages to turn into the mind's rich display of meaning. It's not as though a bean knows how to paint a Madonna and Child, or as though a cauliflower can build the Parthenon.

Every day it's up to you to convert the soul's energy into the meaning of your life. There's no such thing as a meaningless experience. Your brain exists to process meaning. One way or another, the light is going to turn into you. It is going to support the vision you have of yourself, if that is your choice. But in the absence of a vision, it can also be funneled into supporting old habits and closed-off beliefs.

Think of your soul's energy being parceled out like the electricity running to your house. Some portion must go to *basic life support*. Your brain needs to regulate the body's various systems to keep you alive. Another portion of energy goes to *routine activity*. Your brain operates to keep the family going, to do your job at the office, and so on. Some energy also gets allotted to *pleasure*. Your brain thrives on pleasurable sensations and tries to maximize those sensations through entertainment, games, fantasy, sexual arousal, and the like.

So far, the analogy between the soul's energy and the electricity that runs a household is pretty close. Most people run their lives and their households the same way, for basic life support, daily routine, and some amount of pleasure. Yet inside a house might live a Picasso or a Mozart, and here the analogy breaks down, because geniuses maximize the soul's energy for other purposes. Meaning becomes disproportionately important in their lives. Fortunately, the supply of subtle energy is as copious as we want it to be. Once the basics of life are taken care of, there's plenty left over to fuel your personal vision and higher purpose.

As you approach each day, consciously channel energy into your vision. Take any quality of the soul and convert it to your own use. These qualities are not mysterious, and all around you people are creating a purposeful life from the soul level. Let me illustrate the wealth of choice that is available to you.

The soul is *dynamic*. This quality can be converted into a life of adventure, exploration, and forward-looking activity. The overriding theme here is *reaching a goal.*

The soul is *loving*. This quality can be converted into a life of romance, devotion, and worship. The overriding theme here is *ever-expanding bliss.*

The soul is *creative*. This quality can be converted into a life of art, scientific discovery, and self-transformation. The overriding theme is *inspiration.*

The soul is *spontaneous*. This quality can be converted into a life of drama, epiphany, and emotional exploration. The overriding theme is *surprise.*

The soul is *playful*. This quality can be converted into a life of recreation, sport, and carefree enjoyment. The overriding theme is *innocence.*

The soul is *knowing*. This quality can be converted into a life of observation, study, and meditation. The overriding theme is *reflection.*

The soul is *ever-expanding*. This quality can be converted into a life of journeys, breakthroughs, and personal growth. The overriding theme is *evolution.*

With these qualities in mind, you can shape the soul's energy into any kind of life you desire. The shaping is never done automatically, and no one can do it for you. I'm not implying that you will make a choice once and for all. At various stages in your life, different qualities of meaning exert an appeal. "Knowing" generally dominates the student years; "loving" dominates during the phase of relationships and family; "playful" dominates in childhood.

Can a life be shaped without resorting to the soul? Such a life would be either unconscious or shortsighted. Of course such lives exist. There are people who totally dedicate themselves to work for its own sake, to materialism and getting ahead, to saving for the future or protecting the present. One can't call these meaningless choices, but they fall short of the soul's potential to inspire. In some cultures a complete life is one that passes through stages of meaning that everyone is expected to fulfill. I'm thinking primarily of ancient India, where four *ashramas*, or stages of life, were assigned to study, family life, retirement, and finally renunciation of the world. Each stage had its specific duties, and the overall goal was to merge the individual soul with the universal soul—in other words, this was the blueprint for a spiritual journey that every person agreed to for many centuries.

In modern society that broad agreement has broken down, and a toll is paid in lives that feel restless, chaotic, and lacking in meaning. But you don't need society's approval to use your soul's energy in a meaningful way—you don't need anyone's approval. The trajectory of your life can follow whatever arc you choose. The important thing is not to waste energy in the many ways we are all tempted to waste it: through pointless fantasy, unconscious suffering, dead-end habits, inertia, and circular repetition. These are the enemies of a purposeful life. Nourish your "light body" by feeding it with meaning. Recognize the quality of the soul that appeals to you, and interact with the potential that wants to unfold.

Step 2. Turn Entropy into Evolution

Your soul offers a future that is a rising arc from this moment forward. There will be no flat plateaus and no slippery slopes to slide back down. Such a future depends on constant renewal. Your vision must remain fresh, and that can only happen if you find fresh uses for your energy. Without constant input from your soul, however, energy tends to wane. People have come to accept that life will wear itself out as they age. But this is hardly inevitable, even if you look at yourself in materialistic terms. As we saw before, the entire universe is a contest between energy that wants to dissipate and run down (entropy) and energy that wants to become more coherent and complex (evolution). The same contest is waged at the micro level, too, in your cells. Your everyday choices tip the balance one way or the other. If you favor evolution day by day, it's completely reasonable for you to evolve for an entire lifetime.

You have a powerful ally on your side, the mind. Mind isn't subject to entropy. When a thought disappears, it hasn't exhausted your capacity for a new thought to replace it, or a hundred new thoughts. The secret to defeating entropy is to build higher and higher structures in the mind. It is these structures that hold back time and shape a future that keeps improving. To grasp what this means, think of any project that takes more than a day to accomplish: a painting, a book, a scientific problem, or a project at work. When you come back to it, you don't have to mentally start over at the beginning. There's a structure in your mind that keeps your prior work intact, which allows you to pick up where you left off.

In Sanskrit there's a special term for mental structures that endure. They are called *devata*. (The word derives from the Devas. Usually translated as "angels," the Devas are actually the builders and shapers of reality. Without the Devas, awareness would never take shape; it would flow like rainwater across an open field.) To the ancient Vedic seers, *devata*'s job is to make sure that creativity is preserved and not allowed to dissolve. You can even multitask, since the mind is capable of building any number of structures at once. And you can shut off your conscious mind—to go to sleep, for example—without anxiety that entropy will blow away your thoughts like dust in the wind. (Everyone has had the experience of waking up in the morning to find that their first thoughts continue exactly where they left off the night before. Brain chemistry cannot explain this continuity, since chemical reactions change constantly, at a rate of thousands per second in every neuron. Yet *something* keeps our thoughts intact and allows them to build on each other.)

Use the *devata* aspect of your mind to build and keep on building. Never-ending creativity is your goal. In practical terms, this means fighting against boredom, routine, and repetition. Find creative openings at every level of your life, as follows:

Family life is creative as long as each person is interested in every other. No one is put into a box with phrases like "You always do that," or "You're so predictable." No one is labeled and expected to behave according to that label. Fixed roles aren't assigned (e.g., rebel, bad boy, good girl, mother's pet, bully, victim, martyr). Everyone is encouraged to be expressive. Nobody is shut down for acting different.

Relationships are creative if both people find new things to discover in the other. This requires that you move beyond the ego. The ego is by nature self-regarding. It looks to itself first and foremost. Even in the most nearly equal relationships, there's a tendency to take your partner for granted because two egos are involved—you have to look beyond not just your boundaries, but theirs as well. The incentive to find something new in your partner comes from your own sense of change. If you want your own changes to be valued, you must see change in your partner. This sets up a mutual give-and-take. Once started, this give-and-take blossoms into the richest aspect of any relationship: shared evolution.

Work is creative when it satisfies the deepest creative center in a person. New challenges are met by discovering new resources in oneself. As most people find out early in their careers, the problem of boredom and repetition is very real in any occupation. Few workplaces take measures to overcome the problem, so the responsibility lies with you. Remain vigilant for signs that you aren't being challenged, and when those signs appear, demand change. Take on more responsibility; don't shirk risks. If your present situation doesn't permit creative expansion, look for another situation that does. The worst thing is to settle for inertia at work, using the excuse that creativity and pleasure are for after hours and the weekends. You will be leaving a big hole in your life, and that makes wholeness impossible.

Your *vision* is the part of your life that encompasses pure possibility. Whatever energy you devote to building a family life, relationships, and work, there is still enormous room left for reaching higher. Build on your vision every day. It doesn't matter what the vision is, but it should reach beyond your normal boundaries. For some people the vision is humanitarian or religious; for others it is artistic. (For me, in an early adulthood overwhelmed with medical training, a young family, and constant financial pressure, it turned out to be spiritual.) However much you cherish them, family, relationships, and work are transient. Your vision is not. It's your link to the long span of culture and civilization. You get to participate in myth and archetype, a world of heroes and quests. If you keep focusing on your vision, you may touch the fringe of eternity. None of these things is possible without a vision, however. As time unfolds, material life recedes. Having a vision provides insurance that a void isn't waiting at the end of the journey. The miracle is that by dedicating yourself to a vision, you are swept up in the cosmic force of evolution itself, which has no beginning or end.

Step 3. Commit Yourself to Deeper Awareness

Imagine that it's a starry night in June after the moon has gone down. Walk until you find a piece of open ground. Lie on your back and gaze up at the heavens. Can you see yourself in that position? Now think this thought: *There is infinity in all directions, and I am at the center of it.* This isn't an exaggeration—it's literally true that no matter where you stand, you are the center of infinity extending in all directions. The same is true of time. At every minute of your life, eternity stretches before you and behind you. Having absorbed those two ideas, it's hard to feel bound by space and time. Yet there's one more layer to add. Close your eyes, go inside, and think this thought: *The silence I experience is the source of infinity and eternity.*

All the teachings of the greatest spiritual traditions come down to that thought. Jesus and Buddha are linked by knowing that awareness is the source of all that is, was, and ever will be. At your source, time depends on you, not the other way around. Every event that occurs depends on you, in fact, because without awareness the universe ceases to exist. Stars and galaxies vanish. Creation is sucked into a black hole. Your awareness makes reality blossom in all directions, and the deeper your awareness, the richer creation will be. If you can live as if you are the center point of reality, with eternity and infinity expanding all around you, you are living from the level of the soul.

It's mysterious that people don't see themselves this way. But it's easy to be convinced by our eyes, which can see only so far. It's easy to be convinced by our minds, which take in only so much information. And it's easy to be convinced by the ego, which tells you that you are a small, isolated individual overwhelmed by the gigantic scale of the cosmos. Fortunately, as awareness extends, it teaches your eyes, your mind, and your ego to change. In practical terms, when you commit yourself every day to deeper awareness, you are asking for new vision, new beliefs, and a new sense of self.

New vision is possible when you stop being tied to the raw data that your senses bring in. People take for granted that their eyes, for instance, are optical instruments being bombarded by light from the outside. Photons strike the retina, which then transmits billions of photons a minute to the visual cortex to be analyzed. Yet in many traditional cultures, this process is viewed as reversed. Sight goes outward from the mind, seeking to discover the world. In other words, sight carries awareness wherever it wants to go. In many ways this model of the senses is true to our experience. If you don't want to see something, it doesn't matter how many photons bombard your retina. On the other hand, if you are immensely interested in seeing, there's no limit to what you can take in. Consider a gifted artist, who can walk through a crowd on a busy city street and see inspiration in every passing face, every shift of sunlight, every angle of the cityscape.

New vision is creative vision, and you can cultivate it every day. There is unlimited inspiration hidden inside everyday things, waiting for you to pull it out. One of the most famous Chinese paintings consists of two peaches sitting side by side. The artist has reduced each peach to a single stoke of his brush. On the surface this looks like the easiest thing in the world to create, and hardly art at all: you just dip your brush in some black ink, and with a twist of the wrist you draw a circle that looks like a peach. But can you do it so perfectly that the peach looks ripe, sweet, and glistening with beauty? Can you also make the viewer feel that you, the artist, are infinitely sensitive to nature? In this famous image, both things have happened.

Now apply this kind of vision to yourself. Can you look at your child or your spouse so that their essence strikes you, intensely and immediately? Can you transmit love in your glance and feel love in return? We all have this ability. Just as you stand at the center of space and time, so do you stand at the center of love. There is nothing you need to do. New vision comes from the awareness of who you are. When you renew your commitment to having new eyes, they will open.

New beliefs follow automatically from seeing things in a new way. A pupil once came to his spiritual teacher and said, "I don't believe in God." The teacher replied, "You will believe in God when you see him. Have you really looked?" The pupil blushed, taking this as criticism. "I have looked very hard, sir. I pray for God to answer me. I look for signs that He loves me. Nothing works. God might as well not exist." The teacher shook his head. "You think God is invisible, so no wonder you don't see him. The creator is in his creation. Go into nature. Appreciate the trees, the mountains, the green meadows. Look with total love and appreciation, not superficially. At a certain point God will notice that you love his creation. Like an artist who sees someone admiring his painting, God will want to meet you. Then he will come to you, and once you see him, you will believe."

You can take this story as a parable or as the literal truth (taking into account that God is as much she as he, or both merged into one). As a parable, the story says that looking with love and appreciation brings out the subtle levels of nature—including your own nature— and as your perception becomes finer, the sacred level of life reveals itself. At that point you only have to believe in what you've personally experienced. But it's also worthwhile to take the story literally. Gaze at anything you love, whether a beloved person, a rose, or a work of art, and you will see God in it. This is inevitable because there are no things outside yourself, and when you learn to gaze below the surface, you will see your own awareness. And your belief system will shift accordingly, because you have found that believing in yourself is all that you need.

A new sense of self dawns when your belief in yourself is secure. We all hold tight to a self-image that is part fantasy, part projection, and part reflection of other people. If the apple never falls far from the tree, the same holds true for our sense of self. Beginning with our families of origin, we have depended on other people to define us. Are you good or bad, loved or unloved, bright or dull, a leader or a fol- lower? To answer those questions, and hundreds more, you accumu- late information from the outside. This gets blended with your own fantasies and wishes. The final ingredient is the projections you place on other people; that is, you use them to measure yourself by. This entire sense of self is a ramshackle construct, but you depend upon it because you believe you must: otherwise you'd have no idea who you really are.

A new sense of self can replace this construct, one stick at a time, as you experience your awareness, go inside, and meet yourself. The person you meet isn't a flimsy construct. Instead you meet openness, silence, calm, stability, curiosity, love, and the impulse to grow and expand. This new sense of self doesn't need to be constructed. It has existed from the beginning and will always exist. Having met the new you, it becomes easier and easier to throw away bits and pieces of the old one. The process takes patience; you need to meet yourself every day. But it's a joyful process, too, because in your heart of hearts you never bought in to the flimsy construct, not completely. There are too many memories of how it got glued together, piece by piece, sometimes by accident, often against your will. Nobody really wants to be no more than what others see. We yearn to be real, and that yearning, if you keep it in mind, is enough. The person you seek is the same person who is seeking you.

Step 4. Be Generous of Spirit

Wholeness can afford to be generous. It feels no lack. However much you give, more will come to you. I think that's the secret behind the adage that "it is more blessed to give than to receive." When you give, you reveal a spiritual truth, that the flow of life never runs dry. People run into trouble, however, when they give on the surface but feel the pinch of lack underneath. Generosity begins at the level of the soul, which never runs out of the two things totally necessary to life: energy and awareness. When you feel secure that you as a person won't run short of those two things, you can afford to be generous in spirit. That is a greater gift to the world than money. The two don't preclude each other. Once you are generous of spirit, giving on any level becomes natural and easy.

In practical terms, generosity of spirit comes down to the following things:

Offering yourself first.
Never withholding the truth.
Being a force for harmony and coherence.
Placing your trust in the flow of abundance.

All of these points fit our overall purpose of giving you a lifestyle that you can pursue privately while creating real change all around you.

Offer yourself first. Here "yourself" means the real you. Offering an imitation version of yourself is tempting, and most people wind up giving in. They play a role that fits into society's expectations (spouse, worker, authority figure, follower, dependent, victim). They follow the ego's demand for quid pro quo, so that every gift is given with the expectation of a return. They stand upon status and income as defining traits. These factors create a false self because they are external. There's no flow from the inside outward, which is what generosity of spirit is all about. There's an immense difference between stepping forward as a benefactor giving time and money, and stepping forward to offer the real you. The real you is open and vulnerable. It feels sympathy with the human condition. It recognizes no divisions between one soul and another.

It can be frightening to offer the real you, but as so often happens, fear gives false counsel. When you offer the real you, you don't become prey to other people's immense neediness, or to their capacity to take advantage. Rather, you become stronger. The false you, being external, is like a flimsy suit of armor, in this case built from a sense of insecurity. Giving up the false you strips you of armor that was an illusion all along. In reality, your body has been using the unstoppable flow of energy and awareness in order to survive. While you were pretending to be closed, your body remained open to the universe. Why not adopt a strategy that's already been proven to work? Align your spirit with the weak, the dispossessed, the wronged, and the children of the earth. By being open to them, you are not offering yourself as a single soul. You are offering the wholeness of spirit.

Don't withhold the truth. When energy and awareness are flowing, the truth flows with them. Whatever is false serves to block spirit at the source. You aren't being asked to stand up for truth with a capital *T*, because absolutes are not at issue. As life unfolds, you can only represent your truth, and it will change over time as you evolve. Consider the truth about good versus evil. To someone who is less evolved, evil feels powerful, frightening, and starkly opposed to good. With more growth, these things shift: there are gray areas between good and evil. But there is also less fear of evil or belief in its power. When a person is highly evolved, good and evil are less important than separation from the soul, and there is trust that in wholeness the conflict of good versus evil can be resolved. Each position has its own truth as felt by each person.

The important thing is not to withhold your truth, whatever it may be. Truth withheld is truth frozen and stuck. Every time you speak your truth, you are advancing your own evolution. More than that, you are showing your trust in truth to prevail. Untruth is aided more by silence than by lies. I'm thinking not so much on a grand scale as on a very intimate one. In homes where there is physical or emotional abuse, where someone drinks to excess or takes drugs, where signs of depression and anxiety are unmistakable but untreated, the rest of the family generally keeps silent. They passively acquiesce to their own sense of helplessness. The vain hope is that the situation will improve on its own or at the very least remain stable. What actually happens is that silence makes the problem grow worse, because silence implies indifference, hopelessness, unspoken hostility, and lack of options. Speaking the truth opens up options. It shows caring. It rejects hopelessness.

Be a force for harmony and coherence. By definition, wholeness is a state of harmony, while fragmentation is a state of conflict. If we weren't divided inside, we wouldn't be fighting wars against temptation, anger, fear, and self-doubt. The soul is a harmonizing influence, and it shows generosity of spirit to radiate that same quality. A friend told me a striking anecdote recently: He was walking down the street in a big city where he was visiting, and on impulse he went into a fancy bakery, enticed by their extravagant window display. The minute he stepped in the door he saw trouble. The bakery manager was screaming at the girl working the counter. She was in tears, and both were so engrossed that they didn't notice that a customer had entered the shop. My friend said that he had a sudden intuition. *I can bring harmony here.*

He turned his back on the argument, which settled down once his presence was noticed. In itself, that is unremarkable. But my friend kept lingering, and as he did so, he centered himself in his own peace—he's been an experienced meditator for many years. He could feel the atmosphere in the shop soften, and although few would believe what happened next, the manager and the girl at the counter exchanged smiles. By the time my friend left, he saw them embracing and mutually expressing how sorry they were. Can your mere presence bring harmony to a situation the same way? The first step is to believe that it is possible; the second is the willingness not to take sides, but to act solely as a peaceful influence, silently if you can, but speaking up if that becomes necessary. At bottom, conflicts aren't about right and wrong. They are about incoherence, the chaotic emotions and thoughts that result from chaotic energy and fragmented awareness. Right and wrong come into the picture as reflections of turmoil; by screaming that you are right, you don't have to admit that you are hurt, confused, and torn apart yourself. Instead of adding to the turmoil, you can bring in peace, not just because it sounds moral and good to do that, but because without an influence of peace, no productive change can occur.

Place your trust in abundance. Wholeness contains everything; therefore it draws on infinite resources. You may find this a tentative truth in your personal life, because no one is supplied with infinite money, status, power, and love. Where lack doesn't predominate, there is still fear of lack to contend with. Abundance needs to be reframed. When you see it as the infinite resources of spirit, your attention moves away from material things. Instead, you trust that there will always be enough of what your soul has to give. Many people fall back upon religious faith—they believe that God will never bring more challenges than they can handle. But this strikes me as simplistic, because when you look around, many people are silently crushed by their burdens and many more are diminished and overwhelmed. In the opposite camp are the spiritual materialists, the ones who measure divine favor by the size of their bank accounts, who declare that God helps those who help themselves. (Beneath the surface, aren't they really saying that God helps *only* those who help themselves? That's true abandonment of faith, because it reduces God to being a cheerleader for the well-to-do.)

I think it's better to leave faith out of it altogether. Abundance isn't materialistic or religious, either. It's about trusting the flow, knowing that wholeness doesn't have holes in it and never leaves a void. You can be generous with anything the soul gives you, and more will flow in. Be generous with sympathy, love, intelligence, truth, and creativity. The more you express these things, the more will be given to you on all levels. At the same time, don't turn your soul into an ATM machine. The flow isn't a straight line from A to B, and when you are generous, there's no guarantee that a result will follow to your benefit. Yet in the larger scheme you will be evolving every day, as the soul, in flowing through you, transforms you at the same time.

Step 5. Focus on Relationships Instead of Consumption

Wholeness depends on relationships that are whole. You cannot be whole in isolation. Relationship is the true test of any spiritual state; otherwise, you might be deluding yourself—your ego could be using the soul to build itself up. That's the point of a famous anecdote from the lore of yoga:

A spiritual recluse has been sitting in a cave high up in the Himalayas where he pursues enlightenment night and day. Finally, after years of arduous discipline, the light dawns, and the recluse realizes that he has arrived at the goal. Overjoyed, he descends the mountain to deliver the good news to the local villagers. When he gets to the outskirts of town, a beggar reeking of alcohol bumps into him. "Watch where you're going, fool," the recluse mutters. Suddenly he pauses, and without a word he heads back up to his cave.

Relationships become whole as you become whole. But the parallel isn't automatic. You must place your attention on seeing untold potential in another person. I was deeply touched by a visit to Cuba a few years ago. Taken around the island by my hosts, I saw street singers and dancers, common in India when I was a child, but they have now vanished. I saw waitresses smiling and flirting with customers in the cafés; a happy atmosphere prevailed almost everywhere, or so it seemed. One day I asked my driver to explain what I was seeing. "We're too poor to buy anything," he told me. "So we have to focus on relationships." It hadn't occurred to me how seriously consumerism undermines relationships. To consume is to be focused constantly on material goods, but also on the distraction they bring, a flood of video games, television, music, high-tech gadgets, and on and on.

It's degrading to define anyone as a consumer. The image of a voracious open mouth comes to mind (and the inevitable process of waste removal, once digestion is through). But I don't want to make this a moral issue. As your soul sees you, you are connected to everything. To be connected means to be in relationship. Beneath every event in the world are underlying threads that tremble like the disturbance of a spider web. We communicate along these strands of love, sympathy, cooperation, community, and growth. When the strands weaken, so do all those things. (As we saw previously, children who spend hours at video games create a shift in their brains, acquiring special motor skills at the cost of social skills—they can zap fifty alien invaders a minute, but cannot relate to real human beings.) Consumerism exerts a hidden toll by shutting off channels of growth. As a substitute, digital culture has come up with networking, which serves to connect people, usually for a mutual benefit. The more linked you are electronically, the more tied in you are to a global community. But there's no emotional bonding or sense of security in a link. Text messaging gets a few words across, but they come from the most superficial layer of human interaction.

If you look at your own life, you can easily measure how much consumerism has encroached on relationship. The questions are not difficult:

Does my family find time to relate to one another?

How together do we all feel?

Do my children manipulate me to get what they want?

Do I placate my children by bribing them with new things to buy?

In our family, do we rush to be alone with computers, iPods, TV, and video games?

Can we have a family discussion about what really matters?

How often do we deal with problems by seeking more distractions?

Do I measure my worth by how much money I have and the possessions I've accumulated?

Is shopping my therapy?

Few people can answer these questions honestly without feeling uneasy. Of course, distractions offer the easy way out, and relationships raise sensitive issues one would like to avoid. But relating is the only way that any two people can share life together. We don't have to add qualifiers like *committed* relationship, *long-term* relationship, or even *happy* relationship. As an emotion or state of mind, happiness can be induced without going to the trouble of relating to other people, and at the best of times asking another person to make you happy is neither fair nor realistic. What deeply matters in any relationship is the level of awareness that is involved.

On the surface, you relate to someone else to feel better, to get what you want, and to share good things.

If you can take the relationship to a deeper level, it exists to share common goals, to feel supported by another person, and to expand "I" to "we."

If you can go deeper still, a relationship begins to dissolve ego boundaries. The result is a real communion between two people, each living into the other.

Finally, at the level of the soul, there is no "other person."

Individuality gives up its claims as the ego surrenders to spirit. At this level you participate in wholeness, and all your relationships are expansions of wholeness.

Experts often say, and everyone seems to agree, that relationships are hard work. That's certainly true at the ego level, because conflict arises when two egos come into contact. But relating at the level of ego is doomed to begin with, because it points in the opposite direction from the soul. Whenever you find yourself working hard to overcome anything in your relationship—boredom, irritation, hostility, intractable opinions, and areas of disagreement—you've fallen for the ego's agenda. Work as hard as you might, you won't be relating, you will only be negotiating. The secret is to realize that relationships exist entirely in awareness. Because you are the source of awareness, you can shift any relationship within yourself. You don't have to ask for, demand, or negotiate change in the other person. I realize that this goes against the grain of counseling and therapy, but keep in mind that people who bring troubled relationships to a therapist are actually bringing frustrated egos; awareness lost out before the first hour of counseling began.

Once you dedicate yourself to deepening your awareness, relationships must improve, because you are sending new energy along the invisible strands that bond us all. The only caveat is that you must not make awareness a private possession, yet another reason to feel isolated. Let the other person have full advantage of your inner growth. This means that any impulse of love is for them. Any epiphany exists to be shared. As you expand, you must transform being into doing. No matter what happens on the surface, however, rest assured that everyone to whom you relate senses your energy. Bonds don't lie. They cannot be faked. Which is all the more reason to find the true level where bonding occurs. Only there do relationships stop being work and turn effortless. Once you make a bond, there's no reason to distrust the other person, because the two of you are one in the only way that matters, by sharing in the same wholeness. Loneliness, isolation, and the restless insecurity of the ego are exposed for what they are—by-products of disconnected souls before they find each other.

Step 6. Relate to Your Body Consciously

We have all been trained to ignore the spiritual value of our bodies. Centuries of programming have fostered the illusion that the body has no mind, certainly no soul. But as we've seen time and again in this book, your body has kept faith with your soul even when you haven't. It opens itself to the flow of life. It sustains every cell through the universe's infinite supply of energy and intelligence. Ironically, the gratitude given to God should rightfully be given to our bodies, which have sustained us more reliably than any "higher" power. Every day, your body consciously tends to you, never losing focus or attention. You can acknowledge this faithful service by consciously relating to your body in turn.

Or, to be more precise, you will be completing the circle. Awareness wants to flow freely from body to mind and back again. Too often, however, the body sends messages that the mind short-circuits. Certain messages frighten us or undermine our self-image. We don't have time to hear the body, or we procrastinate because there are more important things to attend to. Consider the following everyday situations:

> You feel a twinge of pain.
> You see signs of aging.
> You feel "not quite right" physically.
> You notice that your energy is decreasing.
> You are uncomfortable in your skin.
> You don't see a match between how your body looks and the real you inside.

There are two ways to relate to these experiences. You can detach yourself from the physical sensations and see yourself as separate from them. Or you can think of physical sensations as conscious messages from one part of yourself to another. The first reaction is the easiest and most common. There's a sense of false security that comes from ignoring what our bodies have to say. You get to choose whether to take it seriously; you choose when and where to pay attention. But in essence you are rejecting your body. Real security comes when you relate to your body as consciously as you relate to yourself. Then pain and discomfort acquire a different meaning. They are no longer danger signals that you want to run away from. They are messages asking for a reply. (By analogy, if you're sitting in a restaurant next to a crying baby, your instinct is to be irritated, and if the crying keeps up, you will probably ask for another table. But if it's your own child crying, your instinct is to move toward the disturbance and try to make it better.)

Relating to your body calls for the same basic attitudes that go into any intimate relationship. Tending to them every day keeps the relationship healthy.

Trust
Consideration
Honesty
Mutual cooperation
Loving appreciation

These are all aspects of awareness. People focus too much on the physical choices that the body presents—whether to take vitamins, how many calories to ingest, how much to exercise. Without awareness these considerations tend to be fairly useless. Your body knows if you fear it; it rebels at being disciplined like a disobedient child; being ignored makes it grow dull and inert. The whole purpose of consciously relating to your body is to provide the kind of foundation that is really needed. After that, you can take any physical measures in the right spirit, and that will bring the best results.

Trust. Real trust is implicit. It doesn't depend on shifting moods.

It doesn't need to be tested or proven. Most people only trust their bodies so far. They anticipate a time when the body will bring pain and the distress of aging. If you are on the lookout for what can go wrong physically, you are relating out of distrust, the opposite of what needs to exist. So reframe the situation. Think of the millions of processes that are being carried out perfectly in billions of cells every second. Compared to that steady, faithful, perfectly coordinated functioning, the few times that the body shows distress are minuscule. It's far more realistic to trust your body than to distrust it. After all, you trust your mind even though it occasionally breaks out in irrational reactions and is susceptible to moods of depression and anxiety. Your body stands by you without asking for any reward, and its steadiness far exceeds the shifting winds of the mind.

Consideration. Your body doesn't demand consideration, but it will reward you amply if you show some. It's considerate to walk away from stressful situations. Stress puts enormous pressure on the body's coping mechanisms, and that includes the stress of loud noise, congested work environments, excessive physical demands, and emotional upset. You may consider it recreation to run a marathon, for example, but you should consider your body's viewpoint before demanding that it obey your desire. Another basic consideration is rest and regular daily rhythms. Instead of waiting until you are too tired to go on, provide rest several times a day to your body—all it takes is a few minutes sitting quietly with your eyes closed. A predictable daily routine for meals and exercise also shows consideration. If you are used to irregular habits, it may bore you to adopt new habits, but if you persist for only a week, you will notice a positive response from your body. It will be more relaxed and at the same time more responsive and energetic. Even the most minimal effort at exercise, such as getting up from your desk and stretching every couple of hours, injects a bit of personal attention into the body. Keep in mind that your attention is a basic nutrient that your body needs.

Honesty. In personal relationships, it's a strain to keep up a false front, and the same is true for relating to our body. In both cases the falseness usually comes down to self-image. You look at your body and want it to match your ego's desire to look good in the eyes of others. People spend thousands of hours at the gym, not for the sake of the body, but to satisfy an ego-ideal of beauty, vanity, strength, and security, and to fit in with someone else's expectations. Body image is a huge problem for many people, and classically women are the most distressed about it. You can reframe the whole problem by comparing your body to the person you love most in the world. Do you really care what that person looks like in the mirror? Do you denigrate that person for not fitting the image of a supermodel, not being at their ideal weight, not having perfect biceps or big enough breasts? Does growing older make that person less valuable in your eyes?

The reason those considerations don't matter is that you are relating to a person, not to an object that must match an ideal image. Now think of your body as a person who is just as intimately related to you. You don't even have to call this person "me." By any name, your body has been relating to you as the most faithful of friends, and once you regard it that way, ego image becomes irrelevant. In short, learn to personify your body, and then you won't be so tempted to objectify it.

Mutual cooperation. You can't expect your body to serve you if you give it nothing to work with. The body of a middle-aged executive isn't out to sabotage him when the man decides to shovel a foot of snow from the driveway. But if he has ignored his heart for years, there is danger in sudden hard exertion, perhaps fatal danger. The key to the body's reliability lies in cooperation: only ask for as much as you have given. Compared with other intimate relationships, your body asks for a fraction of what it is willing to give in return. This is another area where it helps to personify your body instead of objectifying it. Think of your body as a willing worker who wants only a meager salary, but who cannot survive on nothing. The salary it asks for is paid in personal attention. If you genuinely want to cooperate with your body, paying it a little attention makes proper diet, exercise, and rest easy—you will be providing those things because you want your willing worker to be happily employed.

Loving appreciation. Your body is going to serve and uphold your interests for a lifetime. It's only fair to appreciate it for this service, and if possible to appreciate it with genuine affection. Most people are far from doing that. Instead they look on their bodies like old models of cars that will need more repairs and cause more trouble as they wear out. This causes a serious disconnect. What they want from life—a future that's more comfortable and fulfilling—is mismatched to a body that grows more uncomfortable and disappointing. The mismatch isn't the body's fault, however; it's the product of beliefs and assumptions born in the mind. We all relate to loved ones who grow older, and if we're lucky, we relate to them better as they age. Familiarity breeds fondness in this case, and appreciation flows more naturally.

The same should hold true with your body. Being a familiar companion, you can grow fonder of it over time. The two of you settle in to a shared life, knowing things about each other that no one else can possibly know. If this sounds like a marriage, that is rightly so. The highest aim in life is the marriage of mind and soul, and since the body links the two, it deserves to be part of a more perfect union as the years unfold. This isn't a fantasy that tries to compensate for the advance of physical aging. It's a realistic way to approach your own awareness. If you aim to be more aware, wiser, and more fulfilled in the future, invite your body to join that future as an equal partner. When body, mind, and soul are matched, the results will be far different from when they are alienated from one another.

Step 7. Embrace Every Day as a New World

For life to turn into a great victory, you have to win many small battles along the way. These are fought on the flat landscape of everyday life. We see the same people each day, by and large, and expect the same things from them. We work according to a routine that becomes

second nature. Lapses into boredom, indifference, and inertia are possible at any time. But beneath this apparent flatness, life is constantly
renewing itself. Your cells are never bored, distracted, inert, or
detached. They are fully engaged in being alive. There seems to be a
gap, then, between mind and body. Since the mind sets the body's
agenda, if you lose the tiny battles against routine, inertia, and boredom, this gap will widen. The flood of renewal will ebb away; forward
motion will gradually come to a halt. If you can close this gap, however, the opposite will happen. Every day will seem like a renewal.

There are two sides to every gap. The model for that is the
synapse, the microscopic gap that separates the branchlike ends of
brain cells. To have any brain activity, chemical messages must leap
across the synapse. On one side is the sender, on the other the
receiver. Both must be prepared to do their job impeccably. When the
synapse stops working, the brain goes out of kilter, which means that
you experience yourself going out of kilter. Your entire sense of self
depends on what happens in the gap. Researchers have discovered, for
example, that depression is linked to how much serotonin, a specific
messenger molecule in the brain, is sent across the synapse and then
taken up again to clear the way for the next burst. In a normal brain
the right amount of serotonin crosses the gap, then just enough is
reabsorbed to keep sender and receiver ready for new messages. In a
depressed person's brain, too much serotonin is reabsorbed, and
with depleted supplies, there's not enough reserve to send the next
message properly. Certain receptors get clogged, and others are
empty. Without the right balance, you can't be in a steady, secure
mood of contentment.

That's a simplified picture, but it says a great deal about how you
meet a new day. Your soul sends energy and awareness, which you are
set to receive. If your brain is occupied with too many old, outworn
experiences, you can only receive a fraction of the new energy and
awareness that is being sent. We all know exactly how this feels. Coming out of a failed relationship, for example, you cannot think about a
new relationship. You aren't receptive on any level, beginning with the

receptors in your brain cells, but extending to your sense of self, what you expect from love, how you view other people, how you cope with disappointment, and so on. It's too crude to think in terms only of molecules crossing a gap. Your whole self comes and goes across the gap, and the receptors that your life depends on are receivers of experience across the whole range of mind and body.

When you woke up this morning, the day could have been entirely fresh. Every day is a new world. Your brain is constructed to receive billions of bits of new data. Nothing compels it to hold on to old experiences that clog up the receiving mechanism. The reason today doesn't feel completely new is that a new self is required. To the extent that you want to bridge yesterday and today with the same old self, renewal is blocked, just as surely as if you tried to fill a brain receptor when it was already full. Under a microscope a cell biologist can see the clogged receptors, and on an MRI a neurologist can point to areas of the brain that aren't as active as they should be. But we must not fall into the trap of thinking that matter controls the self. Your brain won't fill any receptors that you want to keep open. If you reinvent yourself every day, you will experience a new world with every sunrise.

Saying such a thing sends up red flags in a materialistic society. Are we saying that depressed patients caused their serotonin imbalance? Did they fail to receive the joy and fulfillment that their souls wanted to give them? The best answer to that is ambiguous, unfortunately. The brain is on dual control. It runs itself automatically, which means that chemical imbalances can build up on their own, and distorted patterns of brain activity tend to have their own momentum. Once set in place, they recur without outside intervention. So it would be unfair and medically false to claim that a depressed patient caused his condition. On the other hand, people do contribute to their depression. To a huge degree, brain activity is voluntary. If you drink too much, engage in toxic relationships, or lack coping skills in times of stress, the result will be depressed brain function. The shadow zone between the voluntary and the involuntary is very hard to define. In the end, each of us lives in both areas and must navigate them as best we can.

Fortunately, the vast majority of control lies with you personally. You can say "I want to be new today," and 90 percent of the work is done. The trick is to say "I want to be new today" so clearly and with such commitment that the message is received with no mistakes or confusion. Two brain cells facing each other across a synapse may act like separate entities, but in reality they are part of the whole brain. And the brain is part of a larger wholeness—you. It makes all the difference that you are both sender and receiver of every message. Most people don't realize this critical fact; they have constructed a world of "me" and "not me." As soon as they do that, all kinds of messages bombard them from the outside, since "not me" includes other people, the world at large, and Nature itself.

But if everything is "me," then all messages are from one aspect of the self to another. The new day that you awoke to this morning is you in disguise. Its fresh opportunities come from a level of the self that is invisible and immaterial; therefore, wearing the disguise of the external world proves very effective. When you hear the phone ring and pick it up, you hear a voice that is "not me." What could be more convincing? But don't be convinced so easily. Every experience this day brought was subjective; it was received, processed, judged, and absorbed by your awareness. Therefore, this day occurred in awareness, nowhere else, and you *are* awareness.

No two people can experience today in the same way. Even one minute cannot be experienced the same way. Because you are experiencing a unique world, it's up to you how any given moment is received, processed, judged, and absorbed. The self performs these tasks, and the quality of the self determines what you get out of life from moment to moment. At a superficial level there is another person talking to you on the phone—a "not me"—but at the soul level one aspect of awareness is sending a message to another aspect.

The present moment is the only place where renewal is possible, since we receive all messages now. Yet there is no special magic in the now. If a great chef puts an enticing meal in front of you, the experience of eating it doesn't depend on being present in the now. All that matters is the quality of the self as it receives the experience. A distracted person will barely taste the meal, a depressed person will find the food unsavory, but someone in love will think the same food is divine. So the now is like an open brain receptor waiting for the give-and-take of the next message.

If you are completely open, your awareness alert and expanded, your mind free of old conditioning, then the now will appear to be magical. In reality, you supply the magic. Once you realize the central role you play, it comes naturally to embrace every day as a new world. All the things that make it seem like the same old world reside in you, and by focusing on your personal evolution you can get rid of them, The fog that conceals the new world will keep lifting, until the time comes when renewal is effortless and spontaneous. That's the very moment when sender and receiver meet in an unbroken embrace.

Step 8. Let the Timeless Be in Charge of Time

We're told that time should be used wisely, but what does that mean in practice? For most people, it comes down to time management. There are only so many hours in the day, and if too much time is wasted, the day is gone before you've done half the things you set out to do. But your soul doesn't see time that way. Its frame of reference is timeless. Therefore, using time wisely means using it timelessly. If you heard someone say, "My life is timeless," you might have assumed that they were deeply religious, and being timeless means being close to God. Or that they lived in a place like the desert where time seems to stand still. There are other possibilities. The person could be devoted to meditation—a Buddhist, for example, trying to escape the prison of time to reach Nirvana. In other words, the word *timeless* has a mystical ring that may make it confusing and impractical: if you are realistic, your time is better spent trying to cram everything into your day that you want to get done.

It's very important to make the timeless practical. If you turn your back and forget that the timeless exists, you are disconnecting from your soul, which cannot be crammed into a daily schedule. So, is it possible to do the opposite and expand your life into a timeless schedule? To approach this question, think about the various ways that time can go wrong. We can use one example that illustrates the hidden trap that time presents. You have decided to go on a dream vacation, a trip to the Bahamas that will be like a second honeymoon. You and your spouse agree that you both deserve a long break, and by leaving the rest of the family behind, you hope to rekindle your relationship. Unfortunately, things go unexpectedly awry. Planning the trip eats into the little spare time that you have, and you begin to resent your spouse for not doing his share. Your flight to the Caribbean is canceled, stranding you for a day at the airport. You arrive feeling frazzled, unable to relax until practically the day you have to return home. In addition, you spend more time worrying about the kids you left at home than reconnecting intimately with your spouse. It's a relief when the vacation comes to an end, and a month later the whole notion of a second honeymoon feels like a distant memory.

The difference between having a good time and having a bad time actually depends on time itself. In this example, the following things went wrong:

Time became too tight and constricting.
Time created psychological distress.
Under time pressure, experiences felt shallow and unfulfilling.
Time didn't accommodate what you really wanted to happen.

If timelessness can solve these problems, it will turn out to be eminently practical, because the same ills afflict each of us every day. To begin with, take the most basic complaint that all people share: time is too tight. Under the pressure of deadlines, with too many demands on our time, daily life becomes a race with too many finish lines that recede ever farther away the faster you run. Time management attempts to solve this problem, but at best ameliorates it. Work will fill up any time you give it. The solution is to live from a timeless place. Only when time disappears is there enough. That sounds like a paradox, but here's the deeper reasoning:

Time isn't separate from you; it's part of your being. At your source, all events are laid out with perfect timing. The beginning knows the end. Enough time is allotted so that you can not only accomplish all that is needed, but the experience of moving from A to B will also be fulfilling. In other words, the unfolding of time is actually the unfolding of the self. Time cannot trap the self, meaning the real you.

Think of your body when you were in the womb. A normal pregnancy takes nine months for only one reason: the full complexity of a newborn child perfectly fits that span of time. If the embryo needs less or more time, birth adjusts accordingly. There is no pressure dictating that nine months is a fixed deadline. In the same flexible way, anything you want to accomplish is packaged with its own inner schedule. Time submits to your desire, not the other way around. If two people read the same book, the important thing is who got the most out of it, not who got finished first.

Once you see that time is completely subjective, geared to what you want out of life, the whole notion of time pressure vanishes. (The British writer Doris Lessing, who won the Nobel Prize for literature in 2007, dropped out of school in Rhodesia at age fourteen and never returned. She once told an interviewer that this proved to be an enormous advantage, because instead of reading the books that were assigned on schedule in high school and college, she was free to pick up any book when and only when it interested her. In that way she got the most out of everything she read, and her life unfolded in sync with the books that absorbed her.) If you are tied to an external sense of time, you miss the whole point of existence, which is not to meet deadlines.

The timeless knows how to use time far more efficiently than the human mind could possibly calculate. We are not even capable of organizing the body's basic biological rhythms, which are so complex and interwoven that they must be left entirely to Nature. But the mind is quite capable of messing up those rhythms. The same holds true for time in general. The mind may arbitrarily decide that there isn't enough time, that time is running out, that things must be done on time, but in reality the timeless takes care of time. Imagine that you casually spend an hour preparing dinner, reading a magazine article, and doing some light housekeeping. Each thing is untimed. You have a vague sense that you want to get food on the table at a certain hour, but otherwise, fitting everything in its place is effortless. You even have space to think about what you've read and perhaps to entertain a daydream or a future project that is only beginning to gestate.

Now take the same situation but add a phone call saying that your spouse is bringing the boss home for dinner. Time hasn't changed, but your psychological relationship to time has. Now you feel pressure, and what was easy to accomplish is overlaid with anxiety. There's no time to read that magazine article, much less time for reflection, daydreaming, or planning a future project. You have lost the element of the timeless, whose first quality is that time is taken care of. When the task of time management is turned over to the mind, the order it tries to impose is crude and unsatisfying compared with the spontaneous organization of the timeless.

To be whole, you must let the timeless merge with time. That isn't a matter of changing our attitudes alone. You need to cultivate deep awareness, because on the surface, awareness shifts constantly as one thing after another claims your attention. A river runs fastest on the surface, but is nearly motionless at the bottom. Approach your mind that way by finding the still, silent depths that open up through meditation. Like a river, your mind's quiet depths aren't detached from the activity on the surface. Every level of the river is made of the same water and moves toward the same goal. But the journey becomes much more comfortable when you aren't tossed about like a drifting leaf.

It's not at all mystical that a river can be still and moving at the same time. There's no reason to find mysticism in the mind's ability to be still and moving at the same time, either. The timeless merges into time as easily as water merges with water. You can experience this personally. When you discover that being still inside removes the pressure of time, it's inevitable that you will reach the next step, seeing that when the timeless is allowed to handle time, you will never run out of time or be tied to any deadline. The timeless brings freedom, a quality that seeps into time and makes you free this very minute.

Step 9. Feel the World Instead of Trying to Understand It

You can't think your way to wholeness, but you can feel your way there. Leonardo da Vinci spent hundreds of hours near the end of his life trying to figure out the swirling patterns in water as it wended its way downstream, but he never succeeded. Flow refuses to be analyzed, and the same holds true for the flow of life. Yet you were designed with awareness that goes far beyond thinking. You can walk into a room and sense if there's tension in the air. You can sense if someone loves you or not. At a subtler level, you can sense if you belong, or if it's safe. These subtle aspects of awareness guide life far more than people realize. It is mainly in their absence that one sees how crippling it can be not to feel the world.

Here I'm thinking of a young man I know who fell in love with a woman and quickly moved in with her. She was also very much in love, but soon a strange vein of insecurity was exposed in her. Whenever the young man went into the other room, she followed. If he tried to read a book, it wouldn't be long before she would ask, "What are you thinking about?" At first he took the question casually and would reply, "Nothing in particular. Why?" But soon the situation worsened. Every five minutes she would ask, "What are you thinking about?" and no answer would satisfy her. The young man had no idea where this obsession came from, but in the end it caused their relationship to fall apart. Only afterwards did he realize that the woman was unable to feel loved. Anytime the young man became quiet—while reading, working on the computer, or doing nothing at all—she had the panicky feeling that he didn't love her. When she asked, "What are you thinking about?" the only answer that would satisfy her was "I'm thinking of you, darling," and yet even if he gave that answer as affectionately as he could, she would still feel panicked five minutes later.

This is an example of someone who couldn't sense that she was loved, which became a crippling disability. If you feel unlovable to begin with, you cannot sense that someone else loves you. A fixed thought blocks your awareness. In the same way, people who don't feel safe cannot be made to feel safe by any kind of external protection. People who feel unworthy cannot gain self-esteem through any kind of achievement. If you look deep enough, all these cases illustrate a disconnect between the self and the world. We project how we feel onto the external world. If you feel unlovable, the world seems loveless. If you feel unsafe, the world feels dangerous. But isn't the world a dangerous place? Aren't we surrounded by unloving actions and widespread indifference? Yes, but these aren't absolutes. Sometimes the world is dangerous, but most often it's not. Love is absent in many situations, but at unexpected moments love shines through the darkest situation. Instead of trying to understand the endlessly changing world, you can feel your way and trust those feelings. Only then will you know what is unfolding around you.

To be whole requires a very specific feeling: *I am enough*. When you feel that, the world will be enough as well. However, if you feel "I am not enough," the world always will fall short. You will harbor a vague sense that you somehow lack a critical ingredient for fulfillment, and no matter how hard you try to understand it, the missing piece will never be found. Many times in these pages I've said that your body is closer to your soul than you imagine, and this is no exception. Your body knows that it is enough. Cells aren't insecure or worried. If they could speak, they would assert the following things with complete certainty:

I am self-sufficient.

I am safe.

I know exactly how to live.

Life fulfills my needs.

I belong.

Cells live the truth they cannot put into words by constantly being self-sufficient, fitting in perfectly with every other cell, fulfilling their role in the body impeccably. With the body as your foundation, you can feel your way to the certainty that you are enough. Perhaps you've seen widely circulated videos of a blind teenager, afflicted with cancer of the eye as an infant, who has invented his own kind of sonar. Like a dolphin, this boy emits a stream of clicks several times a second and listens to the echoes they make as the sound bounces off objects. In this way he moves with uncanny grace through a dark world. The boy rides a bicycle on his own, plays basketball, and performs household chores. If he is walking down the sidewalk and senses an object blocking his path, he can focus his clicking and "see" that the obstacle is a trashcan, which he then walks around. There are a handful of other sightless patients in the medical literature who have made this adaptation. Apparently their self-created sonar allows them to form mental pictures made of sound.

Only there's a catch here. The sonar used by dolphins— technically known as "echolocation"—requires incredibly fast sound pulses, up to 1,750 clicks per second. A blind person could emit five clicks per second at best, not remotely enough to form a mental image of objects in the near vicinity. How, then, does a sightless person see? One answer is that the body has eyes that are not eyes, primitive areas of the brain just above the spinal column at the base of the skull. Without being connected to the visual cortex and to a pair of eyes, these cells "see" by sensing the outside world directly, the way primitive, single-celled animals steer toward the light. Little is known about "autoscopic vision," as it has been labeled, but this may explain the popular notion of having eyes in the back of your head—you literally do. (Reliable experiments have shown that subjects can sense when someone is looking at them from behind, for example.) The most uncanny examples are people who see their own bodies standing in front of them. Neurologists have recorded a handful of subjects with this kind of vision. When someone has a near-death experience and reports rising up in the air and looking down on her dead body, some kind of autoscopic vision may also be responsible.

These examples don't explain away near-death experiences, or blind people who can see; they show instead that awareness extends far beyond what we generally assume. The body is designed to be aware above and beyond the five senses. If you don't believe that this is true, your mental attitude can block out the subtle awareness that is meant to guide you. On the other hand, you can accept that subtle awareness is real, and once you do, feeling your way through the world becomes a critical part of the spiritual journey. To go back to the woman who kept asking, "What are you thinking about?"—if she had possessed self-awareness, she would feel the panic underlying her obsessive question. Tuning in to this feeling of panic, she would become aware that she felt unloved, and then she would plumb that feeling and conclude that at bottom she feels unlovable. Now a turning point has been reached. She faces a choice. Either being unlovable is a fact that the world keeps cruelly reinforcing, or it's something she can heal in herself. If she makes the choice to heal herself, the cure is to reconnect with her deepest awareness—her soul—which is the source of feeling lovable.

In place of "I am unlovable," one can substitute "I am not safe," "I am not fulfilled," or "I have no purpose." Any sense of lack can be traced back to disconnection from your source. Therefore you can feel your way back and heal the breach. The soul's entire existence depends on the certainty that it is enough. Being whole, nothing can exist outside it. As you reconnect to your soul, feeling your way step by step, your awareness will shift. You are sensing who you really are. "I am enough" is the goal of all spiritual seeking. The good news is that because it is your natural state, your search for wholeness—if you stick with it—is destined to succeed.

Step 10. Seek After Your Own Mystery

Wholeness is yours if you want it. People want jobs, cars, houses, money, and families. They get those things because they go after them, and society is set up to make that possible. But society isn't set up for getting wholeness. Everything spiritual has been put into a separate box from material life. It's true that some people have such strong religious convictions that they want to live a Christian life or a Jewish life or a Muslim life in every respect. The advantage of devoting yourself to religion is that a ready-made path is provided, along with a strong support group. The problem with devoting yourself to religion is that it demands conformity, and if you conform so well that you become the perfect Christian, Muslim, or Jew, there's still no guarantee that you will be whole.

There is no escaping two facts: you must want wholeness as fervently as you want a job, house, car, and family, and you must be willing to walk the path alone. I was deeply moved when the private letters of Mother Teresa were published, years after her death, and the "Mother of Calcutta" revealed that she had never experienced God. Despite her decades of devoted service to the poor, and going against her public image as the perfect saint, Mother Teresa didn't achieve what she wanted—personal knowledge of the divine. For many, this was a depressing revelation. If a saint couldn't reach her spiritual goals, how can we? I'd like to suggest that the answer lies in seeking your own mystery, not one that is handed to you by anyone else. The Buddhists express this by saying, "If you meet the Buddha on the path, kill him." What this means is that if you find yourself trying to conform to a preset ideal, put that notion out of your head.

The mystery of life is your mystery to solve. Every step of the way, you must proceed without preconceptions. It's quite a trick to maintain your passion without a fixed goal in sight. It's so much easier to say to yourself, "One day I will be perfect," or "One day I will meet God, and He will love me." If you pursue a fixed goal, however, you will be like a railroad train whose wheels are held between two rails, unable to move right or left of its own volition. The ability to move in any direction at a moment's notice is critical. Life doesn't come at us along railroad tracks. It comes at us from all directions, and for that reason we need complete freedom of movement, which implies complete freedom of choice. If you have a passion for freedom, that will be good enough at every stage of the spiritual journey.

This was vividly illustrated by a recent experiment with mice that sought to discover how they experienced happiness. Animal researchers define happiness in mice as a brain response. When a mouse is eating, certain areas of its brain light up, indicating contentment and satisfaction. Later, if the mouse is merely reminded of food—through a smell, for example—that is enough to light up the same areas. The situation is similar for human beings. When we are given signals that remind us of being happy (not just the smell of food, but also pictures of loved ones or movies of a beautiful tropical beach), the happiness areas in our brains light up.

Yet here a mystery arises. When a mouse is reminded of happiness, it seeks to increase that response; the smell of food makes it hungry and it wants to eat. Human beings don't pursue happiness in such a linear, predictable way. In terms of the brain, perversity makes no sense. If there is a happiness response, the natural thing would be to light it up as often as possible. Pigeons in cages will keep doing the same task a thousand times if it rewards them with a peck of food. Humans, on the other hand, go without food because we can override biology. A poor mother gives up her dinner so that her child can eat. A political idealist like Gandhi fasts to stir the conscience of his nation's British oppressors. A supermodel subsists on crackers and lemons to conform to the shape that allows her to keep her job. In all these cases the word *perverse* might come to the mind of a brain researcher viewing the situation, but a better word is *transcendent*.

We override biology to go higher, to fulfill a vision of happiness that transcends the happiness we have today. Eating is a biological necessity, but transcending is a human necessity. For us, happiness improves when it has more meaning, purpose, intensity, and wholeness. For millions of people, those things are supplied by their jobs, houses, cars, money, and a family. But if you imagine that you will be perfectly fulfilled once you have all of them, there's a surprise in store for you. The moment you achieve any plateau of satisfaction, a new horizon will open, and your desire to reach that horizon will be as strong as any desire you've ever felt.

That, ultimately, is the mystery. Human beings can never be satisfied with limited fulfillment. We are designed to transcend. As much as you might try to ignore the yearning inside you, it cannot be stifled. You will seek a better kind of happiness, and in so doing, you will be seeking your own mystery. It is that mystery which pertains to common humanity. It brings you up to the level of Buddha and Jesus, and brings them down to your level. The same yearning to transcend unites you, your soul, and every soul. Therefore, you will never have to ignite your passion to be whole. The passion is in you already. It is your birthright.

CONCLUSION:
"WHO MADE ME?"

L ife moves forward by asking the right questions. The first question I remember asking (which my children asked me in turn) was "Who made me?" Children are naturally curious about where they came from. Children take creation personally, as well they should. Yet in their innocence they get steered in the wrong direction. They are told that God made them, or that their parents made them, without revealing the truth, which is that none of us really knows who made us. We have taken one of the most profound mysteries and dismissed it with clichés. We shrug and pass on the answer our parents gave us.

The truth can only be found by exploring who you are. After all, "Who made me?" is the most intimate and personal of questions. You can't know where you belong in the world unless you know where you came from. If you believe the religious answer, that God made you, you will have certainty but no useful knowledge; the mystery of life has been outsourced to Genesis, and the book is closed. This is why people who want useful knowledge have turned to science. Science holds that creation is random, a matter of swirling gases exploding at the moment of the Big Bang. This view at least gives us an ongoing creation. Energy and matter will continue to produce new forms for billions of years, until an exhausted universe has no more energy to give. But a huge price is paid for choosing scientific knowledge. You no longer have a loving, caring Creator. Like every other object, your body is an accidental product of drifting stardust that could just as easily have been sucked out through a black hole. There is no ultimate meaning to life, and no purpose except the ones we make up and fight over.

I have never been able to accept either answer, and my doubt gave rise to these pages, where I've offered a third way. I have tried to reclaim the sacred nature of the body, which is like a forgotten miracle in its exquisite order and intelligence, while supplying useful knowledge of the kind science seeks to find. To uncover that knowledge, we've had to cross over into the invisible territory where materialism feels uncomfortable. But although such things as awareness, intelligence, creativity, and the soul are unseen, this should not delude us into dismissing them as unreal. They are real to us as humans, and that's what counts in the end, because the mystery we want to solve is our own.

I hope the arguments I've made for reinventing the body in terms of energy and awareness come through to you as credible. I believe them fervently, as I believe in bringing the soul back into everyday life. But in the back of my mind I hear myself asking, as I did when I was four years old, "Who made me?"

It is with this, the simplest and yet most profound question, that a spiritual adage comes true. *The journey is the answer.* To find your creator, you must explore the universe until he (or she) appears. In ancient India it was held that all creation was compressed into a human being; therefore, to explore the universe, you needed only to explore yourself. But if you are an objectivist, you can turn the other way and explore the outer world. Following every clue, you will be led eventually to the last frontier of creation, and then you will be overwhelmed by awe. Albert Einstein declared that no great scientific discovery has ever been made except by those who kneel in wonder before the mystery of creation. Wonder is a subjective feeling. Even if you turn outward, you wind up confronting yourself—a blazing galaxy is wondrous only because human eyes are gazing upon it, and the need to understand our wonder is a human need.

Earlier I quoted an old guru who said that the best way to meet

God is to admire his (or her) creation so intensely that the Creator comes out of hiding to meet you. This is rather like an artist who hears about someone who loves his paintings with unbounded enthusiasm. What artist could resist meeting such an admirer? There's a trick to this simple fable, of course, because anyone who has explored Creation to the point of going beyond light and shadow, good and evil, inner and outer, has connected with God already. At that point you and your creator share the same love. Then the only answer to "Who made me?" is "I made myself."

We can allow for the howls of outrage from those who read blasphemy in the idea that human beings created themselves. But no one is usurping God's privileges. The level at which we create ourselves is the level of the soul. The soul is your sacred body. It is the junction point between infinity and the relative world. In that regard I disagree with Einstein. I don't think human awareness must stand in awe before infinity. The thinking mind may be forced to do that, but where thinking fails, consciousness is free to go on. Thinking never invented love, desire, art, music, kindness, altruism, intuition, wisdom, and passion—in fact, all the things that make life worthwhile. When the thinking mind halts in awe before God's creation, love has light-years yet to go; desire still reaches out for more. The process of reinventing the body and resurrecting the soul is a journey, and the journey never ends.

Acknowledgments

In this book I wanted the reader to grasp that life is a process. That truth sinks in when a book is being produced. The process needs an astute and sympathetic editor like Peter Guzzardi, who knows how to steer errant chapters back on the right track. In many ways he is the silent author of the final manuscript. This book crucially needed the supportive environment provided at the publisher's by Shaye Areheart and Jenny Frost. Without their belief in the printed word, my writing would never be allowed to serve a higher purpose. Just as necessary are the people who tend to the details of production and who make an author's life easier from day to day—in this case, Tara Gilbride, Kira Walton, and Julia Pastore.

Thanks to all of you, and as always to Carolyn Rangel, the trusted right hand who always knows what the left hand is doing.

Index

About the Author

Deepak Chopra is the author of more than fifty books translated into over thirty-five languages, including numerous *New York Time* bestsellers in both the fiction and nonfiction categories.

Visit him at www.DeepakChopra.com.